OBSERVATIONS, RUMINATIONS & REFLECTIONS
of a country barber

Once over Lightly

To my DEAR "AUNT" ALICE,
OF WHOM I HAVE THE MOST
FOND MEMORIES OF YEARS PAST.
— Buzz Helm
"TEE BAR"

Buzz Helm

Once over Lightly

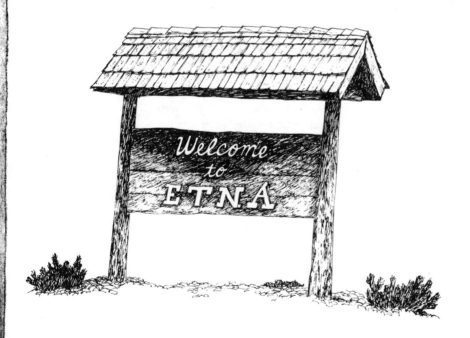

Welcome to ETNA

Illustrations by John D. Jenott

SKETCHBOOKS

SKETCHBOOK PRESS
P.O. Box 220, Fort Jones, CA 96032-0220

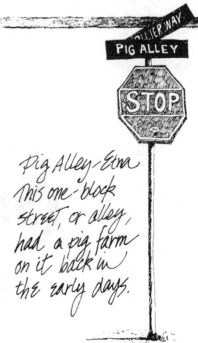

Pig Alley-Etna
This one-block
street, or alley,
had a pig farm
on it back in
the early days.

Once Over Lightly
Observations, Ruminations and Reflections
of a country barber.
By Buzz Helm

Book Design and Illustrations by John D. Jenott

Library of Congress Control Number: 00-090832

International Standard Book Number: 0-9700301-0-X

SKETCHBOOKS

P.O. Box 220, Fort Jones, CA 96032-0220

CONTENTS

OBSERVATIONS

RUMINATIONS

REFLECTIONS

FOREWORD...and FOREWARNED

Wrinkles should merely indicate where smiles have been.
                                                        Mark Twain

Mark Twain said it, so it must be so. Which means that this book might give you a few wrinkles: **FOREWARNED.**

Every Wednesday I read Buzz Helm's column, "Once Over Lightly," in our weekly newspaper, the *Pioneer Press*. It is an enjoyable read: full of humor, nostalgia, and a quizzical look at life's endless foibles—always good for chuckles and smiles (more wrinkles according to the estimable Mr. Twain).

However, over time it became clear to me that this was more than a enjoyable read... I found that after a lifetime of working as an illustrator, these essays would invariably create humorous pictures in my mind as I read them.   With this enlightened awareness I approached Buzz with the idea of putting together a selection of them in a book with my illustrations.

Buzz didn't exactly do cartwheels of joy, in fact he looked pretty doubtful about the whole venture. I believe he was thinking about my book, the *Scott Valley Sketchbook*, and wondering how that kind of representational art could possibly work with his light-hearted (mostly) essays. He certainly could not have known that I had had considerable experience in cartooning and animation.

Now Buzz had been my barber for quite a spell, so after thinking about it for a few minutes he finally said, "Well, I've always found your head to be fairly sound. There are a few odd-ball bumps here and there, but on the whole your skull seems reasonably thick. So if you want to do it, why I'll dig out some ol' columns and get them over to you."

That's how it got started, and, as the popular country song says, "That's my story and I'm sticking to it."

It has a happier ending than the song.

A Bit About Buzz...

There are several ways
You can go through this life.
You can laugh,
You can cry,
Or you can sit there
With a sour face,
And watch this life go by.

Personally, I prefer to laugh.

Welcome to the inner world of Buzz Helm's head. To say that Buzz sees the world slightly askew from the rest of us is like saying that Marilyn Monroe was of the female gender —slight understatement.

My Thesaurus gives the synonyms to "Buzz" as "hum, drone, whir, hiss, whizz." I don't know about hum, drone, hiss, but certainly whir and whizz.

My theory for Buzz's oblique view of life is that he has been a barber for some 50 years—which means that for over a half century he has been talking to the backs of heads, or in the mirror, which puts his client in reverse image.

I'm not sure, but it seems to me that this might affect a person's outlook on the variables of life—but like I said, this is just a theory.

However, and this is a fact, after nearly 30 years of cutting hair in Scott Valley, Buzz recognizes the guys more readily from the back than from the front. This was confirmed one day when, in a crowd, a voice behind me said, "Hello, John." I turned around and there was Buzz —whir and whizz— strange.

Whatever: If you prefer to laugh, read on. You may not go, "haw, haw, haw," it's a gentle humor (mostly), but you certainly are going to nod your head in agreement and chuckle. And according to modern medicine, chuckling is good for your health. So read on, chuckle, be healthy, and live a long and happy life — laugh.

John Jenott, Fort Jones, CA, Jan. 2000

Dedicated to Jeanne, My "ELW" — *Buzz*

In December of 1978, Gary Mortenson, Editor and Publisher of Scott Valley's weekly newspaper, the *Pioneer Press,* asked me if I would write a gossip column for the paper. I agreed to try, and the first one was printed on January 3rd, 1979. It was called simply the "Etna Column." Three years later he asked me if I would do a humorous column each week in addition to the "Etna Column," and I agreed to try it.

The first one was printed on October 6th, 1982, and was called "Once Over Lightly." I have continued to do both of these columns since then and have turned in over 1,018 "Etna Columns," and over 928 "Once Over Lightly" columns, and am still trying. Some of my friends will testify to the fact that I am trying...very trying.

It was only through the constant encouragement of my ever loving Jeanne.... My "ELW," that I was able to crank out these once-a-week helpings of brain barf.

The idea of publishing some of them in book form was the brainchild of my friend, John Jenott, who did the artwork and the putting of it together.

Here it is then. I hope you enjoy it.

Buzz Helm, Etna, California, Jan. 2000

6

OBSERVATIONS

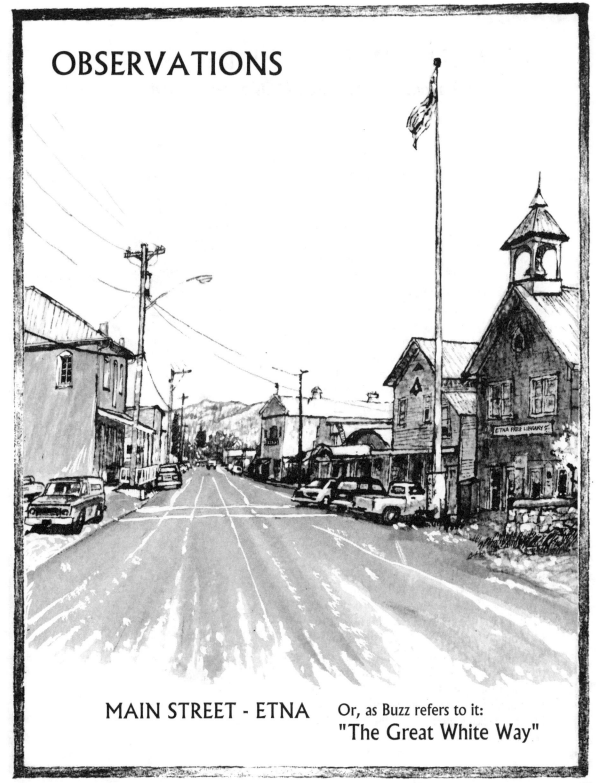

MAIN STREET - ETNA   Or, as Buzz refers to it:
"The Great White Way"

THE WONDERMENT OF KIDS

Think about it — we were all kids once; how did we survive it?

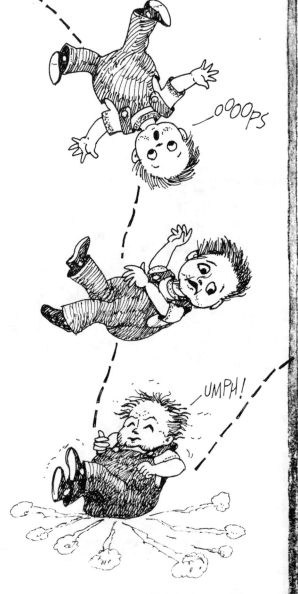

....One of the wonders of the world must certainly be none other than kids.

Now, I realize that some people are offended by the term 'kid' being applied to children. So, out of respect to those few, I offer these alternate terms: "curtain climbers," "rug runners," "linoleum lizards," and "tricycle motors."

By any name you choose to call them, they are still a most amazing machine. They have the ability to fall off a 5 foot high porch, land right on their little punkin' and bounce around like three-day old Jell-O without busting any bones or tearing any vital organs loose.

One time while I was waiting for my ELW (ever lovin' wife) at a shopping center I saw all kinds of things happen to kids.

I just sat there in the safety of the car and observed various tumbles and falls that these little guys took without requiring the services of an ambulance or paramedics.

At least three of them, in the time lapse of about 45 minutes, fell off a mechanical pony that just rocked back and forth. The mom would get involved in a conversation with a friend and not pay any attention to the young'n and there he would go, right off the rocking pony onto the nice hard concrete.

One got his foot hung up in the rein when he fell and was in such a position that every time the pony rocked it bounced his head on the hard metal base of the contraption.

Oh sure, they cry a little bit from being scared and a twinge of hurt, but by golly, they don't break anything.

Parents themselves trust this factor I guess. They jerk them around by one arm with the feet off the ground and give 'em a few whacks on the legs and seat...it looks like the kid's arm rotates a full 360 degrees but it doesn't come unscrewed.

Others were sandwiched in between rows of shopping carts with just their arms and legs visible, at first glance you'd swear the body part had been completely demolished and cast aside somewhere on the asphalt. But nope, just mad cause he dropped his ice cream cone.

They are a wonderment in other ways too. They have a constant problem with nose juice running onto their upper lip and come equipped with some unknown sticky substance all over their hands, and when this stuff is in full bloom they get that uncontrollable urge to hug a grown-up around the neck, right after the grown-up has put on a fresh white shirt.

They can find a greasy or dirty spot to roll in...always right after they have been all shined up to go someplace.

I think they could get all dirtied up like that even if they were turned loose in an operating room in the cleanest hospital in the world.

Yep, they are a most amazing little outfit, and the meanest man in the world can feel his heart melt a little bit when one of these lil' creatures looks him right in the eye, smiles and wants to hold his hand....Awww shucks.

April 30, 1984

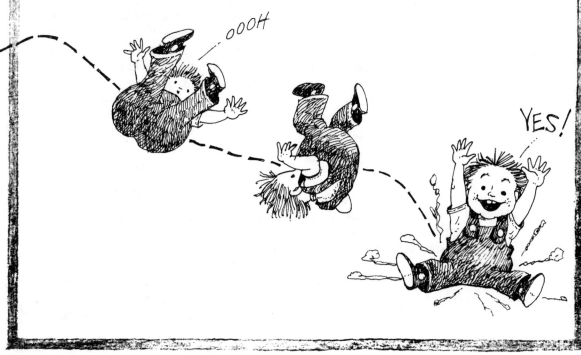

THE EVOLUTION OF SODY POP

A look at the world of endless fizzy flavors

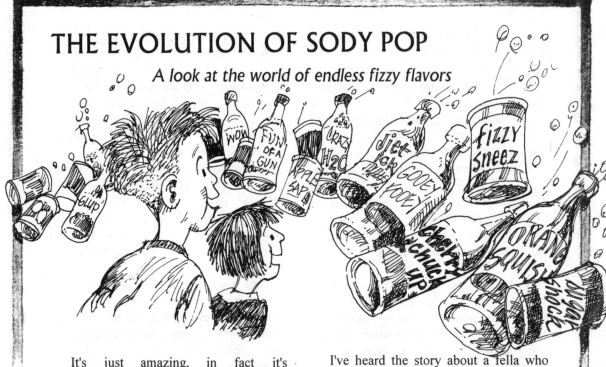

It's just amazing, in fact it's awesome...the number and brands of all the different soft drinks that are on the market these days. We, the people, are either drinking one heck of a lot of this stuff or some of these companies are not making much money.

I just don't see how they can all be selling enough to remain in business. Do you suppose it's possible that all these outfits could be owned by one company and they just act like they compete with each other?

Back in the old days (I hear tell) there was only one soft drink that was sold on the premises and it was sarsaparilla, usually called "sassprella". It was made from some sort of a root and was said to be overly sweet tasting and not too good as a thirst quencher.

Later on it became known as root beer when they started putting the fizzy stuff in it.

I've heard the story about a fella who grew up to the ripe old age of 22 without ever having tasted any kind of a soft drink and just barely knew what the stuff was, never having ever ventured any further from the farm than the swampy south forty. Anyhow, the draft got him in 1942 and the guys in the barracks got him to try a Coke and asked him what he thought of it. He took another long drink of the stuff, gasped for air and wheezed out, "It tastes exactly like it feels when my foot goes to sleep."

I was in the third grade of grammar school when I took my first slug of soda pop..."Shet 'em up agin barkeep, lesh keep 'em comin'."

There were a lot flavors of Nehi sody pop...grape, orange, lemon, cream, etc. Of course there was Coca Cola or "Coke" as it was called, even then. There was a nasty rumor going around, probably started by the competition, that made hints that Coke was just that — that they used cocaine in the recipe and it wasn't good for you to drink it. Somehow the Coca Cola people were able to put down the rumor and really made a firm stand as the number one seller of sody pop...orr maybe it was because of the rumor that they were such a big success.

Then Pepsi Cola came out to do battle with the Coke people. They offered a bigger bottle of sody for the same price and had a jingle to advertise the fact..."Pepsi Cola hits the spot , twelve full ounces that's a lot, twice as much for a nickel too, Pepsi Cola is the drink for you, nickel, nickel, nickel."

It was maybe one of the first singing commercials. Then Royal Crown Cola came along to knock Pepsi out of the ring. "RC" they called it and that was about it for the soft drinks as near as I can remember...just a few to choose from.

There was also some stuff called "near beer" that was sort of sold as a soft drink...kids could have the stuff. It had the taste of beer, but there was no alcohol in it, although it foamed and had a head on it. As a fella said once, regarding near beer, "The guy that named this stuff near beer was a darn poor judge of distance."

It didn't take all day to decide which kind of sody pop you wanted then...and every store didn't carry all the kinds either. One thing they all have in common though...they are all fizzy and make your innards feel as if you've swallowed a Fourth of July sparkler while it was lit.

August 7, 1980

SHET 'EM UP AGAIN, BARKEEP...

11

ALWAYS WEAR CLEAN UNDERWEAR

Save yourself disgusting embarrassment...
Mom's admonition is still valid today.

It's funny sometimes the way things will run through your mind that you haven't thought about for years. Once in a while it's just a part of a conversation that triggers the ol' memory. Along about the time that a lot of us were kids ('bout a millyun years ago) it was a common thing for mothers to want the kids to wear clean underwear in case they were hurt in some kind of accident and hauled to the hospital so the doctor wouldn't exclaim, "M'gawd, look at this kid's dirty underwear...we can't work on him."

I always thought to myself that when I grew up and became rich that I would wear bran' new underwear every day so that I would get the very best of medical care if I was taken to the hospital in an unconscious state.

Of course there was always another way of thinking about this thing...on days when a kid didn't have on clean underwear, he was extra careful about everything, trying to cut down on the possibility of becoming injured in some kind of accident.

On days when he had on fresh underwear, he was reckless and devil-may-care as if he was safe from embarrassment of being taken to the operating room with dirty shorts and tee-shirt.

These things stay with some of us for a long time. Not too long ago the evening news on TV was showing a film of a fireman making a daring and dangerous rescue attempt to save a person from a burning building with no regard whatsoever for his own safety. I thought to myself, "That guy must have on some really nifty underwear." He had no fear of getting taken to the doctor.

In today's world of modern medicine this has ceased to be a factor. To insure that everyone gets the same medical attention, regardless of the condition of his underwear, an orderly takes away all your clothes before the doctor ever sees you...that guarantees fair and equal treatment of all patients.

There were lots of other things that you had to be careful about too. Such as if you

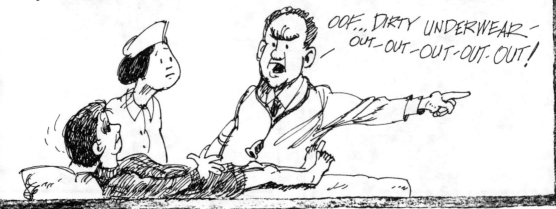

OOF... DIRTY UNDERWEAR - OUT-OUT-OUT-OUT. OUT!

were going to get treated to a new pair of shoes (a rare occasion) you had to be sure to wear that one precious pair of socks...the ones that didn't have holes in 'em, so the guy in the shoe store wouldn't refuse to sell you some shoes 'cause your toe was sticking out of your sock.

I'll bet a lot of us remember this one..."Clean up your plate, kids in Europe are starving." To this day I wonder how many European kids I saved from starvation by eating everything on my plate.

May 5, 1982

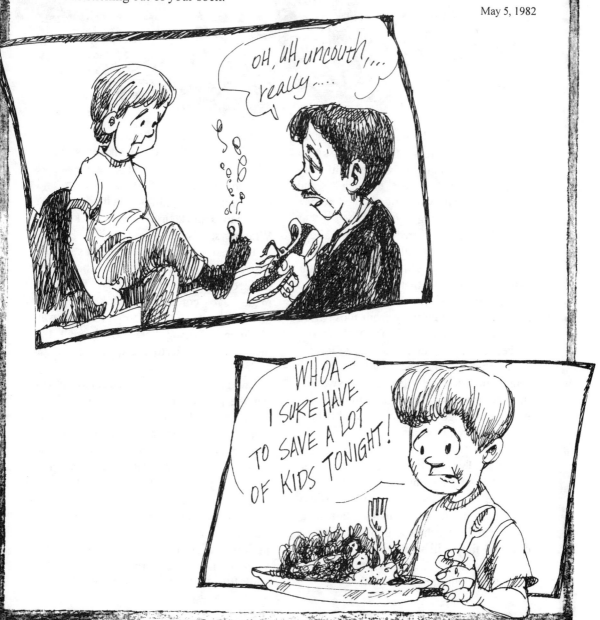

13

GOING TO THE FAIR
...and the dangers thereof

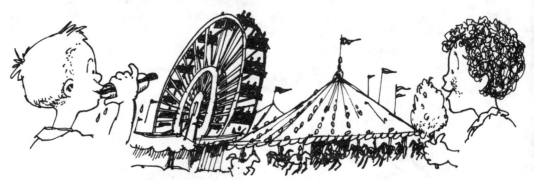

Gosh, what could be a better way to spend a day than visiting the Siskiyou County Golden Fair. It's a wonderful way to get out in the heat and enjoy the overwhelming crowd of overheated human bodies all crushing against each other along the fairway, orrrr "cholesterol alley" as it is sometimes called by the senior citizen community....All those food booths hawking everything that tastes so good and is so prohibited by the doctors that care for the seniors. "Stay away from those fried hamburgers" and "Don't eat those barbecued beef sandwiches" and so forth.

In other words, the word is for the seniors that if it tastes good, don't swallow it....Spit it out; it can't be good for you. It's better if you go down to the rabbit barn and share some alfalfa pellets with the bunnies.

I know I've mentioned this before, but it's a strange phenomenon that kids under the age of six are born with a sticky substance on their lil' hands and face. They can be washed a hundred times a day, and they will still come up with that secret formula gooey goop that is ever present on their upper extremities.

One fair season I remember I was strolling along the main walkway and had this odd sensation that something was sort of holding me back. I looked down, and there was this cute lil' kid behind me with both hands stuck firmly to the back of my Wranglers.

The really odd thing is I wasn't sure just where I picked him up, and he hadn't noticed that I wasn't his daddy. When we made eye contact, I think we both screamed out loud. Not too far behind was his mama forcing her way through the heavy foot traffic to get to him or us or whichever.

I was convinced that I would have to cut out the part of my pants that he had his hands on...either that or take the pants clear off. A fella in a Pepsi Cola booth was eyeing the whole affair and he shouted over, "Come get some ice and rub it on the junk and it will peel off." By golly he was right.

I said he must have a few kids of his own to know a trick like that, but he said he wasn't even married....He had just been working fairs and carnivals most of his adult life and learned a few tricks like that.

I think the stuff was diagnosed as a combination of candied apple and cotton candy with a hint of caramel corn for more binding.

If you are lucky enough to find a bench to sit down on and rest a bit, be sure to look before you sit. Always expect to find a wad of bubble gun or a half devoured burrito lying there in wait for a victim.

I have to say though, the ELW (ever lovin' wife) and I have usually been able to find a grassy spot in the shade behind the buildings and off the main walkway where we can sit and enjoy a bag of popcorn (no butter, no salt) and a nice cold drink (Diet Coke or Pepsi) and watch the human parade from afar.

I don't want to sound like I'm knocking the fair. I think it's a great event, and I realy enjoy the exhibits and livestock. I just kind of thought I'd bring up some the natural pitfalls that plague any popular public event, and the fair is a very popular event.

I would miss it a lot if it ever didn't happen. Keep it up, Ron. You're doin' great!

August 13, 1997

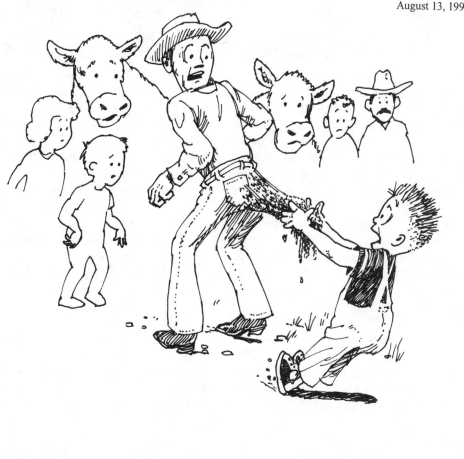

15

WE WERE SO POOR...

...and other tear jerkers

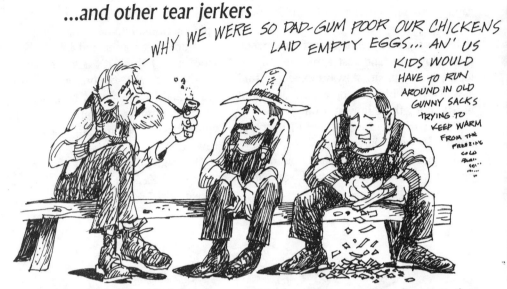

WHY WE WERE SO DAD-GUM POOR OUR CHICKENS LAID EMPTY EGGS... AN' US KIDS WOULD HAVE TO RUN AROUND IN OLD GUNNY SACKS TRYING TO KEEP WARM FROM THE FREEZING COLD AIR...

It never fails...this time of the year always brings out the old "poor boy stories." You know what I mean,..."When I was a kid we were so poor that..." One of the many things I really like about being around a good old "man's" barber shop is the way the conversations go...the theme changes and the topic varies but the stories just keep right on flowing.

One fella was saying that one Christmas Eve, when he was a kid, they all heard a shogun blast out in the yard and their dad came in the house looking real sad and he said, "I feel so bad....I just shot Santa Claus by mistake; I thought it was a big chicken hawk....I guess there won't be no presents this year."

The guy said he found out years later that his dad just did that 'cause he had no money for gifts that year...too poor, so he made up that story and shot the gun in the air.

Another fella was telling how one time he got new shoes for a present and then the next year he got the box that they came in...he was supposed to use the cardboard to put inside and cover up the holes in the soles of the shoes he got the year before...(sniff-sob).

The next guy says, "When we were kids things were so bad, no money in the family, we'd hand down clothes at Christmas. There was four of us kids and one year mama said it was time to trade our underwear for the Yule Season. Me, Tom and Fred didn't mind too much, but Elizabeth just hated the whole idea." (choke-gurgle-snurk).

Next...."Well sir by golly, you know we didn't always have a great big feast on the table, but by shucks we got by....One year mama gave us dried apples for breakfast and for lunch we got warm water, then for dinner we'd just swell up." (oh woe-schlurg-sob-blub).

16

Next...."Now, round about the time I wuz thirteen years old we was eatin' Christmas dinner and I reached for a second slice of fried mush, my ol' daddy said, son ain't you ever gonna get out on yer own and start buyin' yer vittles fer yerseff?" (oh boo-hoo snuff-glurg).

Step right up...."There wuz seven of us kids and our clothes were all tattered and shredded, just held together with the holes. When we'd run in the wind they'd make a sort of hummin' sound and we got so we could run in formation and make it sound sumpthin' like organ music...folks would toss coins to us and that's how we got enough money for a baloney roast on Christmas." (aahgg-blubber-sob wheeze-snurf).

Lemmee try one...."Us kids were all real skinny and gaunt, but we'd really have to watch lil' ol' Ephram, if we didn't wash all the possum fat off him after Christmas dinner, the dog would think he smelled like scraps and try to bury him in the yard." (cough-gag-slub-sob).

As for me, I'm not gonna try to add anything to those above, I'm too choked up and watery eyed, but I will say, in closing, I'm happy that my brother and I didn't have a sister around underwear tradin' time...lucky girl, that not sister of ours.

December 13, 1989

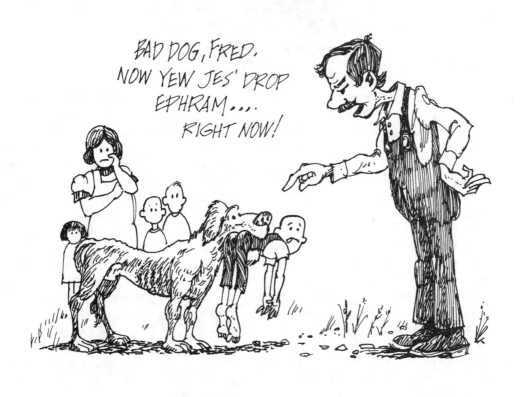

BAD DOG, FRED. NOW YEW JES' DROP EPHRAM.... RIGHT NOW!

AH......YOUTH!

they just keep gettin' younger

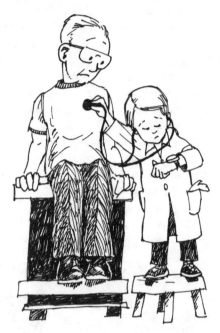

Y'know, I'm more conscious of youth than I should be now that the people in charge are suddenly looking younger and younger; people like doctors and congressmen and policemen. How can you be comfortable when your blood pressure is being taken by someone who looks like he should be asking to borrow the family car?

Not too long ago I was at the Medford Clinic to see a specialist, and after I had been placed in one of those little crypt rooms and was sitting on the table with the paper cover, a kid came in and said, "What can I do for you?" He looked like a kid who worked at Taco Bell a few weeks before, so I said, "Thanks, but I'm waiting for the doctor....How long you been working here?"

He told me he was the doctor and had been there about three years. Oops...awkward feeling...humada, hubada stutter, stammer...."Sorry doc, you look so young." He said I couldn't hurt his feelings by telling him how young he looked, aaaand at my age I should be able to understand that real well.

You have to admit there is something just a little unnerving about watching the evening political news and seeing some kid with zits and a yo-yo tell about some bill he is going to author to present at the next legislative session.

Something about bringing skate board parts under governmental scrutiny....Too many flat-wheeled skateboards on the rental rack, or something like that. I don't know....Weird!

I was way down south in Red Bluff last summer at the cafe stop and two police cars pulled in, one policeman in each car. They had evidently been in radio contact and agreed to meet there for coffee and pie.

When they got out of their black and whites (Holstein cars), I saw how young they were, and I fully expected them to go into that hand slappin' thing...you know, "Gimme a high five, now low on the slide, now two on the cross, way low bro." but they didn't. They acted very adult. They sure could have passed the "graduation plus one summer" age.

Now that I look back I can understand a lot of stuff that happened and was said to me when I was of tender age....F'rinstance,

when I reported to the Platoon Sergeant and told him my orders were to report to him as a replacement he said, "Holy jumpin' horn toads! How old are you kid?" I pulled myself up to my full five foot ten and replied, "I've had my 17th birthday awhile back."

He shook his head and went off mumblin' stuff like, "If he's 17 I'm 102....If they send 'em to me any younger I'll be orderin' pablum and teethin' rings."

Anyhow, examining the situation, I guess I'm happy that all those professional people and civic leaders and law enforcement people are not my age...........
I guess.

December 11, 1996

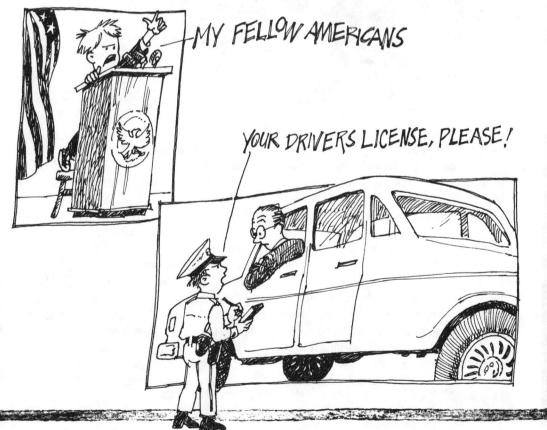

19

RODEO!
not to be confused with lawn croquet

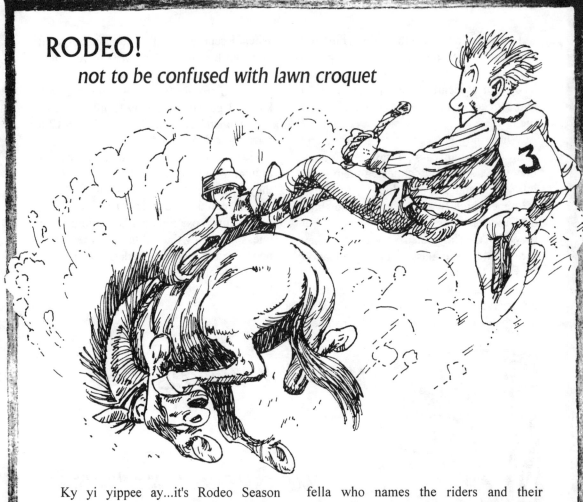

Ky yi yippee ay...it's Rodeo Season again! Red Bluff Round Up was last weekend and the rest of 'em just follow right along one after the other. The best show on earth and the roughest sport there is, that's rodeo. Whether you want to call it a "ro-dee-o" or a "ro-day-o" you have to admit it's a spectator sport that leaves no dull spots.

Now, there is one highly technical and specialized job at a rodeo that requires snap decisions, quick wit and the ability to take the crowd's mind off an unfortunate mishap in the arena. That one person is none other than the rodeo announcer, that fella who names the riders and their opponents as they come out of the chute gates or as they enter the other competitions.

He has to be able to make light of a bad injury or an accident to keep the crowd from choking on their hot dogs. One of the guys I always think of when the "big money" rodeos are going on is Rex Allen.

Rex could always come up with something to say that would sound like he had been rehearsing it for a week, and deliver it in his slow western drawl so that you never missed a syllable, such as..."Well looky there, that ol' bronc is tryin' to get right up there in the saddle with that cowboy an' he says if you're gettin' on, I'm gettin' off...an' my oh my he lands hard right on his wallet."

The translation of this verse is, the bucking horse got his hind hoof stuck in the stirrup, did a front summersault and landed right in the lap of the cowboy who had hit the ground in sitting position. The arena clowns hauled the whole mess away in a couple of gunny sacks.

Getting closer to home, I have to say that Ron Lillard does a fine job of announcing such as, "I do believe that ol' bull bent his neck around and scratched that cowboy with his horn. Did he get ya Roy?"

Roy manages a wave as he picks up his hat, hoping that's where he will find his head, and also both sets of ribs are neatly dovetailed together over on his left side.

Right here at home there's a fella who does a real fine job of announcing and is definitely a local favorite, an' that's Mike

Bryan. Now Mike might say something like this during a real muddy cowhide race, "Did ya notice the rooster tails behind that hide rider when they hit that biggest wallow out there?"...translates into, when the guy on the hide ducked his head to keep from eatin' an iron horse shoe (still attached to the horse) the mud went down inside the front of his shirt, into his Levis, forcing his boots off and allowing the mud to squirt out both pants legs in a sort of jet action like the wake of the high-powered speedboats which travel about the same speed.

As for the riders themselves, I think about the only thing they're scared of, is not being able to walk out of the arena under their own power; they'll make it to the back of the chutes an' then collapse in a heap, neatly covered by their contestant number which has floated down and landed on top.

April 20, 1983

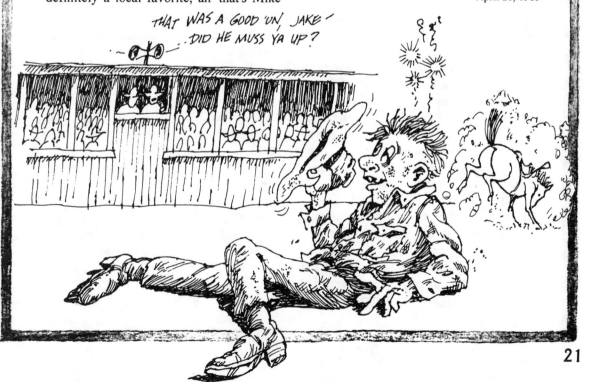

21

ON THE ROAD
obey the speed limit? good luck, podner.

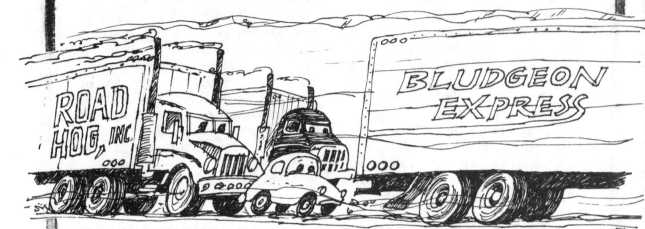

Having just returned home from a trip south, I'd like to highlight a few things I notice about getting on the ol' "concrete ribbon" that we call I-5 South...aaaand, coming home we call it I-5 North. I always end up having a few names of my own that I like to call it, but I'll spare the tender ears of some and hold my tongue in check.

To begin with, I do not like, repeat, do not like to run in the truck lane. It's rough, full of holes, and the trucks travel that lane. I also like to stay within the speed limit that is designated for the several different sections of the freeway. Some places it's double nickel (55) and some places it's 65 and still in others it's 70.

Now the problem I have is, if I'm traveling at 55 mph, the traffic gets right on my bumper, and the guy behind me starts flashing his lights and giving me those hand signals that are international sign language, so I pull over in the truck lane. Jiggle-jiggle bump-bump and thump.

Before I get an opening to get back in the left lane, my rear view mirror fills up with a big radiator that has "Kenworth" written across it in big letters.

As near as I can tell, the cars are going at least 70 mph in the left lane, and the trucks are going 65 mph in their lane which leaves no place for the guy that's trying to obey the law and drive 55 mph.

As a person gets in the other different speed zones, the problem stays the same. The faster the limit, the faster the traffic goes. Down there in the olive country around Corning, I was just keeping up with the flow of the truck traffic since I was in the truck lane. I couldn't keep up in the car lane.

I happened to look down at the big gauge and the needle was bumping 73 mph, and my mirror was completely filled with big letters that said, "Mack." I could even see the bugs stuck in the fins of the radiator.

I told the ELW (ever lovin' wife) that I

was gonna see if I could get some tranquilizers the size of English muffins for the return trip and just pop 'em like M&Ms.

Occasionally you can spot a Holstein car (CHP) sitting on an overpass watching the flow. As long as nobodys driving crazy and cutting in and out, they don't seem to mind the speed they are going. It's the flow that counts, I guess, smooth and even.

There is another thing that bothers me. I have no complaint about cars driving daylight hours with their headlights on, even when there is no fog or smog, but why is it they think they have to have the high beams on?

In some cases they have not only the high beams on but the extra set of driving lights on too, making in all four bright lights coming at you. The low beam would accomplish the same result. They would be seen, and that's the point, I think.

I overheard a trucker one time when the subject was about the daytime high beams, and he said to his buddy, "Y'know Smokey, a handful of marbles takes care of the lil' problem if ya learn jest when to toss 'em. Timin' is everything."

Here's wishing all of you, friend and foe alike, a very Happy, Healthy New Year, and remember, keep your sense of humor. Have a good one!

December 31, 1997

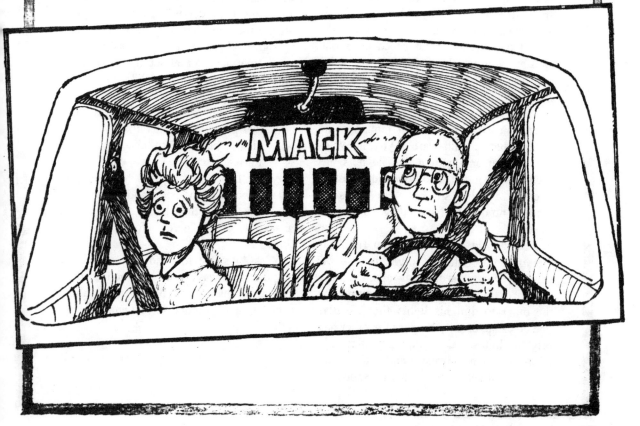

ON THE ROAD...AGAIN
etiquette, road rage, stress and ulcers

I don't do an awful lot of driving down I-5, or any other major highway...just a few times a year, but it's interesting how the same people games have been going on since Highway 99 and lil' ol' two lane strips, and probably long before that.

You know what I mean about games....F'rinstance, and I know this has happened to most of us at one time or another; say that the guy ahead of you is driving about the same speed as you are and then for some reason begins to gradually slow up until you have no choice but to pass him. Well, he will probably do one of two things, either speed up about the time you get along side of him, or he will pass you immediately after you have gotten around him.

I like the routine where he speeds up when you get along side of him...he will pretend that he is unaware of you, he won't look at you or anything, but he puts the "pedal to the metal" and now you're lost in a cloud of blue smoke. He utters to himself, no doubt, "Now I've got you, you (bleep)."

The age old practice of "you first" on dimming the lights at night is a good game. Two fellas meeting along a long stretch of highway, each one waiting for the other to dim his lights first...finally, one gives up, usually because the other has brighter lights. Orrr, one guy dims his lights well in advance and other one doesn't, just keeps 'em on high. Sooo, the first fella waits until the bright one is real close to him and pops 'em bright and just leaves them there hoping that the guy's eye pupils are shrunk down to the size of pin heads. "Now I've gotcha you (bleep)." A real extreme case of headlight "get eveness"...maybe one guy has been following another fella for a long time at a pretty close distance with his brights on, shining right in the rear glass and flooding the whole cockpit with brightness. So what happens?...The first fella either slows up so the behinder will pass, or he pulls off the road and lets him go by then pulls in right behind him and gives him the same treatment for about the next thirty miles.."take that you (bleep)."

Passing up a hitchhiker can have some interesting spin off happenings....If you have ever passed up a hitchhiker, and it's a good idea to pass 'em up, check your rear view mirror after you've gone by. You may see the fella standing there holding his cardboard "LA" sign and giving you the most interesting hand gestures...real unsavory stuff..."here's for you, you (bleep)."

Yesss, it's just too bad that everybody on the highway doesn't practice their driving etiquette and be as polite about everything as you and I...you and me...us? Whichever.

October 23, 1985

24

THE OL' PICKUP TRUCK
the country gentleman's favorite

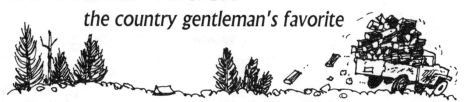

Y'know...there is probably not a more versatile, all 'round handy, easy to like and hard to get along without vehicle, than...a good ol' pickup truck.

If a fella had a dozen different rigs on the place and somebody told him that he was only allowed to have one...betcha he'd pick the pickup to keep.

Consider the "half ton" pickup f'rinstance. Heck, if you can't pile 25 or 30 bales of hay on that sucker, you just aren't trying.

If you own a "three quarter ton" pickup you ought to be able to put on about 2500 pounds of wet crushed serpentine with no effort at all...and the only thing that puts a limit on the amount of firewood that you can pile on is the inability of the average guy to cut and split that much wood in a morning.

Pickups very definitely have their own distinctive markings that indicate what line of work their owner is involved in, like...a pickup that has all four fenders crushed and a couple 50 gallon drums in the back with dust sticking to spilled oil and diesel on the tailgate and a package of Beech Nut or Copenhagen laying on the dashboard, it's a logger.

If a pickup has a bunch of used bailing wire piled in the back and an almost completely demolished tailgate and a package of Beech Nut or Copenhagen laying on the dashboard, it's a cowboy.

If a pickup is a four-wheel drive with a bent up Barden Bumper and a shovel and a pair of rubber boots in the back with a package of Beech Nut or Copenhagen laying on the dashboard, it's a farmer.

If a pickup has a rack on it that goes clear out over the cab with a big tool box in the back and has paint and/or cement splashed on the hood and a package of Beech Nut or Copenhagen laying on the dashboard, it's a building contractor.

If a pickup shows several of, or any combination, of any the above mentioned features, but does not have a package of Beech Nut or Copenhagen laying on the dashboard then it probably belongs to a one vehicle family and it gets used for everything.

If you ever see ('twould be a rare sight indeed) a fella washing his pickup...he's either a tourist, a man bored out of his mind, or a guy getting ready to trade his pickup in on a new one and wants it to look as good as possible when he goes to make a deal..."Hey, whattyaknow...this pickup is real purty blue. I never could remember what color I bought last time." Well, that may be stretching it a little, everybody remembers what color their pickup is, shucks...at least I know mine is a sort of green, or gray...or ummm, maybe brown, orrr red? Maybe I better wash it.

March 24, 1982

THE TELEPHONE SOLICITOR

What the heck!
When you get that annoying unwanted call, you might as well have fun.

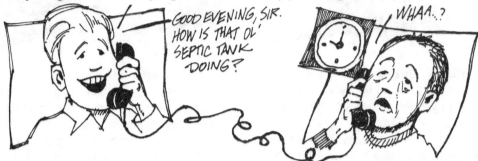

I suppose everyone has to make a living some way or other, but I have to say sometimes I get just a little upset with these telephone calls from folks who are trying to sell something...especially when they call after 10 o'clock at night.

Once in a while these guys will catch me in a weird mood, and I'm just enough out of sorts that I turn kind of mean and sorta play with these calls a little bit....I always hate myself in the morning though.

F'rinstance, and maybe a lot of you got a call from the same outfit, this call came at about 10:30 at night.   I answered, expecting it to be a relative with some sort of bad news or something....The voice asked, "Hello, Mr. Helm?" Wellll, I knew by the "Mr. Helm" thing that it wasn't a relative or friend or even a casual acquaintance and I felt this playful mood crawl up the nape of my neck.

I said, "Nooo, Mr. Helm was my dad and he passed away quite some time ago. I'm Buzz Helm." The voice gave me a name that I didn't quite get, but it didn't matter...."Well Buzz, this is not an effort to sell you something. I just want to ask you a couple of questions."

I braced myself, fighting down rudeness and told him to go right ahead and ask his questions and said in the most rural voice I could muster, "I sure do hope I got the right answers.   I like contests."   He explained that it wasn't a contest, and there were no prizes involved...."Is your home on a septic tank?" he asked.

I said, "Shucks no, what kind of a fool would build his house on top of a septic tank....There's a septic tank pretty close to the house though, maybe 15 or 20 feet away"....I went on, "Y'know, I was thinkin', in order for a house to be on top of a septic tank they would have to put in the septic tank first and then build the house wouldn't they?"

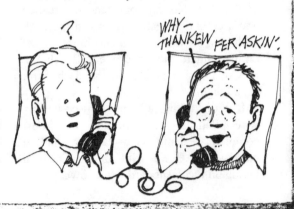

He said, "I'm not sure about how they would do that...I just wanted to know whether or not your home was connected to a subscriber service." I told him that I did subscribe to a couple of magazines and a local newspaper and that if he was sellin' magazines he was wastin' his time, I didn't want any more.

He said, "No, no, I meant I wanted to know if you used a septic tank or a sewer service." I explained to him further, "My septic tank is my sewer service, and since the tank was there I'd be a durn fool not to use it, wouldn't I?"

He agreed that made sense all right...he guessed. He said, "What I want to know is, do you ever add anything to the tank to increase its action?" I fought down my first inclination for an answer and said instead, "I ain't never seen no action to the septic tank, it just stays in the same spot all the time...very calm and gentle."

I heard him kind of sigh and take a deep breath. "Has your tank ever gotten full and had to be pumped out by a septic tank service?" I told him the tank had been in the ground since about 1899 and to my knowledge it had never been full because there was an outlet near the top that drained it into the creek when it got that full, so it never could get clear up to the top of the tank and concluded with, "Am I gettin' any of these answers right to the questions?"

He said, "You've done just fine Mr. Helm, I mean Buzz, and I've got to hang up now.... Many more calls to make you see."

I still think that darn guy was trying to sell something, but he never got around to it.

January 26, 1994

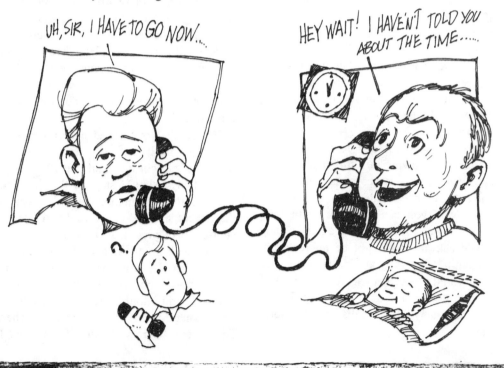

UH, SIR, I HAVE TO GO NOW...

HEY WAIT! I HAVEN'T TOLD YOU ABOUT THE TIME......

THE TELEPHONE SOLICITOR - AGAIN
they're taking the fun out of it

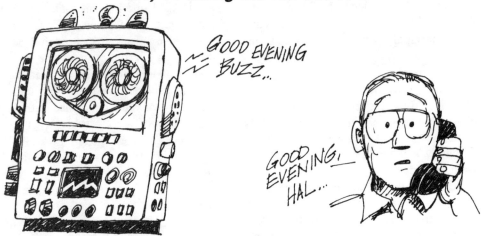

GOOD EVENING BUZZ...

GOOD EVENING, HAL...

Well now they've done it! Part of my recreation used to be jerking these telephone solicitors around when they call me...especially those late night ones...the after 10 p.m. ones. I especially make it a point to make their call interesting for them.

Anyhow, the last two calls that I've had are recordings. Yes, recordings! Now how in heck are ya gonna yank a recording around? The latest one was for siding on my house. The recording said this was a recording made for people who may be interested in having this stuff put on their house, and if they were, to stay on the line and listen to the recorded information.

No way you can have fun with that. When it used to be a real live person they would ask me if I might be interested in something like that, and when I said no they would proceed anyhow. I know...all I have to do is hang up, but, shucks, I don't get that many phone calls and it's sorta fun.

When they'd ask me what type of existing siding I had I would tell 'em dumb stuff like, "Oh, I've got bark on there right now, you know that stuff on the outside of trees." Then I would sometimes go on to say, "Yep, before the bark we used to collect old car license plates and nail 'em on but that was when everybody had to renew their plates every year and there was lots of throw aways...not too many these days."

Before that one I had a recorded call from that outfit that sells stuff for septic tanks. The recording said that if I used a septic tank I should stay on the line and listen to the information. Wellll, darn it, there went another one. I used to tell these septic tank guys that I never had any trouble with my tank...I lived right next to a year round stream and I just had the whole house on a eight inch pipe that emptied right into the stream, gravity flow. "You can't do that!" they'd exclaim. Then I'd tell 'em, "Sure you can. If you want I can send you a diagram showin' just how we did it. It was easy."

Maybe it was guys like me that caused 'em to start with the recording thing. Last August I got a late night call from a fella who started out with, "Just what did you do today to save an endangered species, any kind?" Welllll, I told him that I didn't kill a whale that day, at least not in the afternoon...an' I hadn't eliminated a mole or gopher for over a week, but as long as I live here they will for sure be endangered.

He began to get a tad upset with my manner, so I told him I had a question for him. Like, what was his outfit doin' to save the slaughter of Naugas. Wasteful slaughter! I don't even know what a Nauga looks like, and I've never seen Naugaburger or Nauga steaks for sale. They must surely just skin 'em and throw the carcass away...inhumane! Wasteful! Yet, they just go on using the hides for commercial purposes. Most furniture and new cars are all upholstered with Naugahyde and that takes a lot of those creatures...maybe two and a half for one front seat.

They try to cover up their dastardly crime by purposefully misspelling the word "hide" to make it "hyde," but there are a few of us who know what's going on! Click!...dial tone!....Why that darn guy hung up on me! I don't blame him. His days are probably tough enough without touching base with guys like me.

November 30, 1994

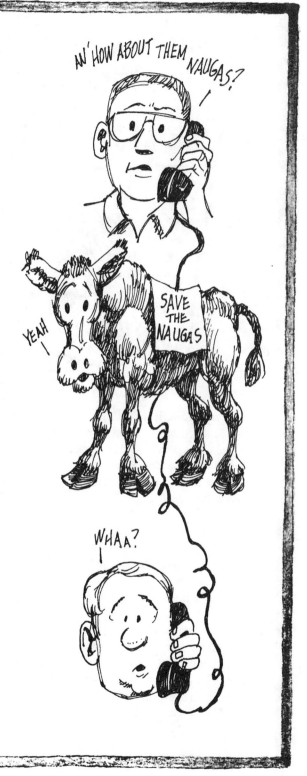

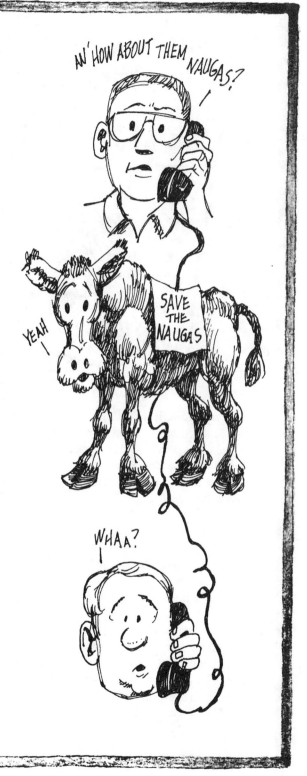

29

GOPHERS AND WOODPECKERS
those dirty little bleep-bleep-bleep-bleep!

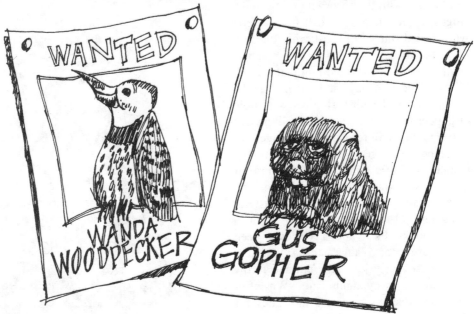

There are only two living creatures on my scatter that are on the endangered species list...one is the gopher and the other is the woodpecker.

They are in danger whenever they make themselves visible.

I just can't understand it...there are thousands of acres of nice big trees out there and plenty of dry dead ones that are much more tasty than mine I would think. They are not satisfied with merely killing my shade trees, they are slowly digesting my house.

I have replaced some of the trim around my second story windows more than I care to remember. One time a feller told me that if I would replace that trim with cedar instead of pine or fir, the woodpeckers wouldn't bother it because the taste was offensive to them. Wrong!!

The primer hadn't even dried completely before there was one up there banging away. It's weird the way the darn things know what your intentions are. When there is one out there with his lil' jackhammer going I can get up very quietly, nice and slow, sneak to the shotgun rack, pick up a couple shells and zoom! He's gone.

That's one reason I sort of look forward to winter each year, the woodpecker traffic slows down a bit. The other reason that winter doesn't seem too bad is that the gopher activity comes to an almost complete standstill.

I thought I had the solution to the gopher problem this spring when a very nice gentleman gave me one of those yard

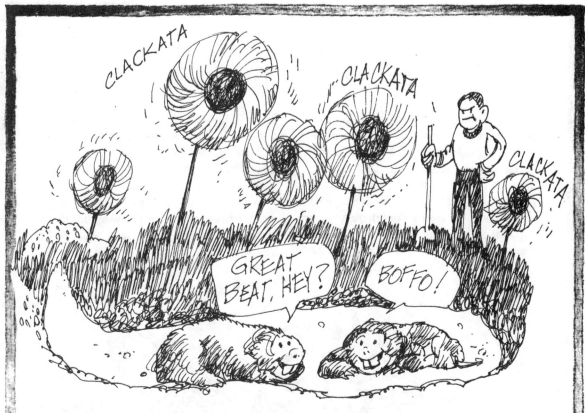

daisy gadgets. I had tried them before and nothing changed but this fella had a better idea...he placed a round of buckshot in the big daisy...when the wind turned the flower the lead ball would rattle and send the noise down into the ground through the wire support that held the daisy in the dirt.

For awhile the gophers gave that thing a wide berth, but, pretty soon they were back raising big mounds all around the noisy daisy.

I've no doubt shortened my own life handling all the poisons down through the years.

I tried cyanide gas bombs, poison grain, traffic flares, poison peanuts etc. I'm considering buying some surplus Army land mines, if I could get some with a trigger that was sensitive enough that a gopher's weight would trigger the thing.

Setting those traps is a no gain play....I make a bigger mess digging a hole to set the things in than the diggers do. I'm convinced that the only solution to the woodpecker and gopher problem is to rent an upstairs apartment on about the 17th floor without even a window box for flowers and nothing but plastic greenery in dry pots and then thoroughly search every person and package that enters the premises...might keep the place free of the lil' monsters...trouble is, Etna has not, as yet, become infected with the high rise mania.

I guess (sigh) I would really rather have the bothersome crittters than that sort of digressing progressing.

October 4, 1989

MORE WOODPECKERS
and more bleep-bleep-bleep-bleep!

It's jest not fair, doggone it! With the whole Klamath National Forest out there for 'em to peck on and make holes in, why do the ding busted muddle-headed, muley brained, cotton-eyed (apologies to Gabby Hayes) woodpeckers have to pick (peck?) on my house? I can't go out there and ruin one of their trees cause they have a sign on them that says " Wildlife Tree, Do Not Cut"...and there are a lot of those signs on trees.

Trees. I found a fella who was willing to replace all those boards and trim. He told me that if they were made out of cedar wood the "woodys" wouldn't bother them 'cause they didn't like the taste of cedar.

Well sir/mam, the paint hadn't even dried before the woodys were up there knockin' themselves out with their little built-in jackhammers so, scratch that rule off the list. Since then I just make it a practice to get up there at about five year

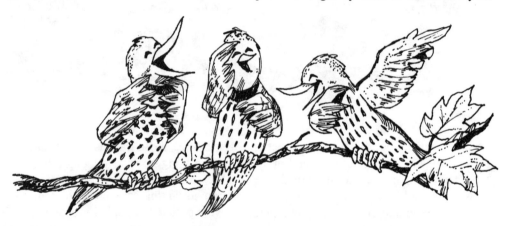

About every five years or so I have to climb up there about forty feet and repair a bunch of holes that woodpeckers have made. It seems to me that they have a special taste for these old two-story house like mine, maybe it's because they know how much trouble it is to get up there and work on 'em.

When the ELW (ever-loving wife) and I first bought this place, every board along the eaves was full of holes. It looked as if the thing had been made out of Joshua

intervals and patch holes with this stuff that you mix up with water, when it dries it gets just as hard as concrete. The way I figger it, in about twenty years (if I survive that long) I should just about have the entire area that they like so much, one hundred percent filled in with this hard stuff and there should be a bunch of woodpeckers flying around with badly bent beaks.

That might make them an even worse menace than ever though, come to think of

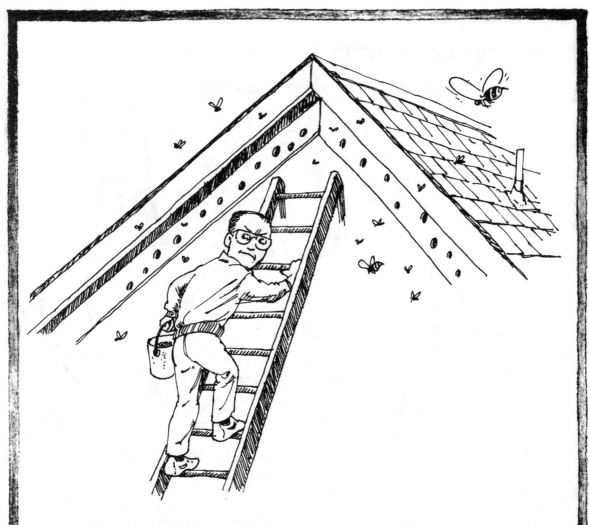

it...with a crooked beak they could hide around the corner and peck on the opposite side; might have to make a new entry in the bird book, such as, "Beakus Curvasus, commonly called Bent Beak Flicker".

This little periodic repair job has some interesting side effects too. Some of the holes go clear through to the attic which makes a fine place for black wasps and yellow wasps to set up housekeeping...and they get real irate when a humanoid starts to fool around with their living space and they attack in squadrons. They come at

you with the speed boards open, full throttle and the landing hook down and locked...whammo!

I'm almost finished with the job for this year...about three more cans of wasp and hornet spray and another five pounds of that stuff that's mixed with water to make patching goop and one more tube of insect sting salve, I'd like to do the job a little oftener, but I figger five years in between that sort of entertainment is about quick enough.

August 21, 1985

CHICKENS UNITE!

giving credit where it belongs

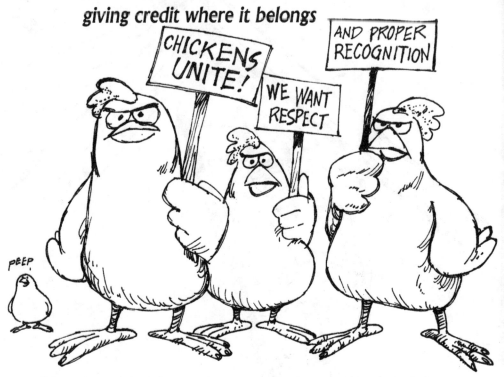

I am speaking this week in defense and support of the American Chicken. The Chicken has for many years been slighted at this time of year. I mean, it's bad enough that they are taken for granted as always ready to sacrifice themselves as a Sunday dinner when nothing else has been planned. F'rinstance, I'm sure you have all heard a conversation similar to this, "What's for dinner today, Hon? Oh, I don't know, why don't you lop the head off one of those chickens?"

Done! The dinner problem is solved.

The chicken is under a great deal of strain around the Easter Season to supply all the eggs that are needed. Think about it. Every organization in America that you can think of has and Easter Egg Hunt.

Kiwanis, Rotary, Lions, Optimists etc. They all hard boil dozens and dozens of eggs to be colored and hidden. Almost every church has it's own Easter Egg Hunt right after Sunday Services. Dozens and dozens and dozens of eggs. I have this vision of the chicken farmer out there all night long in the hen house with his whip, lashing the poor creatures and hollering, "Faster, more eggs, more eggs, Easter is almost here!"

The worst part of the whole thing is that the rabbits get all the credit for supplying all these eggs. Step up and ask any lil' kid, "Where do all these eggs come from?" and the young'n will reply without hesitation, "The Easter Bunny brought 'em." Now, all rabbits at Easter time are automatically considered to be Easter Bunnies. Walk up to any rabbit and ask, "How many Easter eggs have you supplied us this year?" The rabbit will not even try to deny that rabbits are not responsible for all those eggs. They just get that sly look on their faces and sort of shrug as if to say, "No big thing, I don't know." If a rabbit had an ounce of decency he (or she) could at least say, "We rabbits do not supply the Easter Eggs, the chickens do that." But noooo, they don't utter a word, just take the credit and roll with it.

Just as a test sometime, ask a child, "Did the Easter Chicken bring a lot of Easter Eggs for you?" The kid will say, "You mean Easter Bunny, there's no Easter Chicken." The chicken gets shot down again.

As Senator Leghorn might say, "Chickens, ah say chickens, we will hafta arise. Ah mean, arise and identify ourselves, ah say identify with the Easter Season or be forever, ah say forever, overlooked. Are ya lissinin' rabbit? Cute kid but he don't lissin'."

Well, no matter who gets credit for supplying the eggs, I never get over the enjoyment I get from watching those lil' kids hunt for and find those Easter Eggs. Every time I get a flashback to when our family used to have the egg hunts in our own yard. The first thing on Easter morning those two lil' critters would get out there and scrounge for those brightly colored eggs. Neither one of our kids particularly cared for hard boiled chicken eggs, but they loved those chocolate ones the Easter Bunny brought, all wrapped up in pretty paper.

March 31, 1999

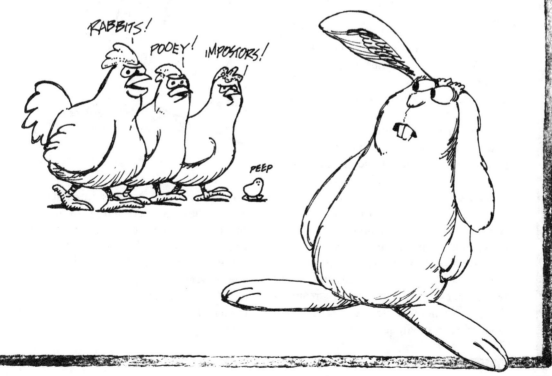

SNOW

and snow...snow...snow...snow...snow...snow...snow...

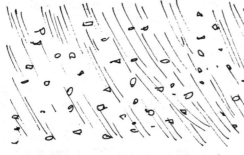

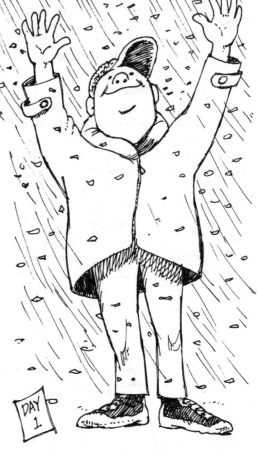

It all depends on how you look at it ...aaand the way you look at it depends on how long you have to look at it. What I have in mind is winter in general and snow storms in particular. Just say f'rinstance that after a long hot dry summer a fella is witnessing the first snow storm of the season...really soaking up the beauty of it, enjoying the clean scene that it's producing. It might go something like this...

"It's just the most awesome thing, experiencing one of Mother Nature's beautiful displays of her might and her power. Look how every flake falls individually and silently into it's own little niche of the scheme of things. You know, they say that there are no two snowflakes exactly the same, each one is different. How silently they build one upon the other creating depth and beauty....how wonderful."

Now the second day of the storm..."It is getting quite deep now and the drifts are going to make it difficult to get out to the main road. It's rather nice though, having this odd sense of abandonment and mildly feeling cut off from the main stream of things...so quietly white and pretty. I ah, I wonder when it will quit?"

The third day...same storm..."It's sure lucky I have a good supply of firewood and plenty of hay, otherwise I'd begin to worry just a tad. The darn stuff has been coming down steady for three days now, it doesn't seem to be quite as pretty as when it first started...must have some Lozangelus smog mixed in with it or something."

On the fourth day..."Well, I'll be a red-headed raccoon (sorry Gabby) it's still snowing about as hard as ever. When is the darn stuff gonna let up! Enough is enough, an' I'm running a little short on grocery items...gettin' down to stuff in the freezer and canned goods. Gettin' tired of kickin' the stupid stuff out of the way every time I step outside...c'mon, quit willya!"

On the fifth day,..."Aw fer...! Will ya look at that...the doggone stuff is still dumpin' down on me. Geez! I wish it would stop just fer a few hours, at least long enough to sorta dig out a bit....I'm sick of it, sick! sick! sick! An another thing, if she (the wife) plays that Christmas record album one more time, I'm gonna bounce the whole machine right off her head. An listen to them ignorant cows, bawlin' their heads off for hay. I ain't never seen anything so all-out ugly as three feet of snow all over the whole place. That's it, I'm through, finished! Come spring this place goes on the market! I'm head'n down to a warmer climate."

Welll, I guess it's all in how a fella looks at it...orrr how it begins to look to a fella.

December 4, 1985

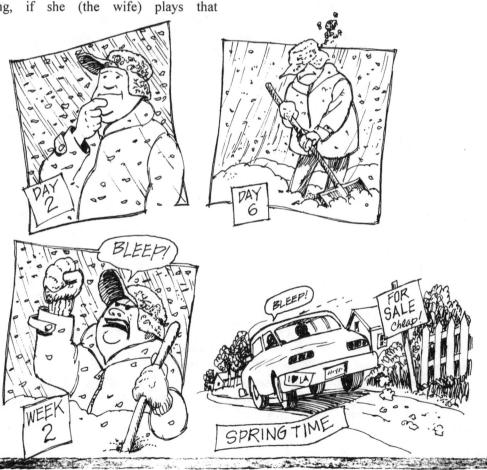

OUR NATIONAL BIRD!

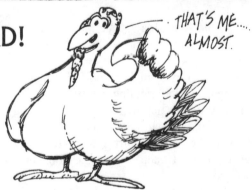

THAT'S ME.... ALMOST.

Here 'tis...almost another Thanksgiving Day holiday is upon us. It is really spooky how fast the years seem to be slipping by. I guess one might call an old timer one who can remember when the stores waited until Thanksgiving had past before they bombarded us with their high-powered salesmanship and covered us up with Christmas ads. Somehow the big guys haven't discovered any way to capitalize on the nation's national turkey day. Of course, the food markets run their ads and sell a lot of food. Shucks, that's what the folks have always done...planned for a big meal and have the whole family together for the day.

Turkey has always been the main thing on Thanksgiving with the rest of the meal planned around the ol' turkey bird. I think it was Teddy Roosevelt, when he was the President, that wanted to make the turkey our national bird instead of the eagle. He considered the eagle little more than a common vulture or buzzard, but thought the turkey had style and grace...and tasted a heck of a lot better. The thing is, if he had succeeded in his endeavor it may have become illegal to eat a turkey. I admit it wouldn't seem right eating our national symbol. If I remember correctly the heart and cholesterol people don't have any quarrel with turkey as long as you don't eat

the skin or the dressing or the gravy or the etc. The rule of thumb with those diets is, if it tastes good don't swallow....It's unhealthy.

Thanksgiving traditionally has been a family get-together day...an easy going no schedule day. A day to reflect on our many blessings in this country that we live in and enjoy the fellowship of relatives and friends.

I think a lot of the holiday meals are planned to coincide with a football game on TV these days. I have trouble remembering what the afternoon's activity was after the big meal before there was TV. Seems like first of all it was a little nap while the table was being cleared and then card games or other games like board games. Canasta was very big there for awhile...just a few short years before TV. For the life of me I cannot remember a doggone thing about how canasta was played. Pinochle was big...cribbage was always my favorite.

I just don't see how any commercialism could improve on a day like our American Thanksgiving Day holiday....Can't think of a thing.

Happy Thanksgiving Day to all of you nice folks out there, and many more!

November 23, 1994

WEATHER (man?)

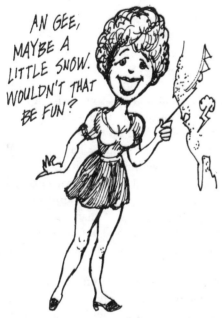

AN GEE,
MAYBE A
LITTLE SNOW.
WOULDN'T THAT
BE FUN?

I have just recently started watching and listening to weathermen again. I quit during all that hot dry summer weather...There was nothing a weatherman could tell me that I didn't already know.

F'rinstance, the evening news on TV usually devotes a sizable part of their news program to a weatherman and his report. Typically one of these fellas spends valuable time telling you how hot or wet or windy it was in your locale on that day. Is that something that belongs on a news program? I mean we were there. We knew how hot or wet or windy it was. What I would like to see and hear from the weatherman is what the weather will be for the next 24 or 36 hours, not what it was for the last 24 or 36 hours.

Weathermen of the past several years have spent more time becoming a "personality" than doing a good job of predicting what we could expect from the elements for the next few hours. Willard Scott is now quite a TV personality and where did he get his start? Reporting the weather on national TV that's where. Each day he would stretch his part a little further, devoting less and less time to the weather information.

In the early days of TV they had what was known as "weather girls"....They didn't know anything at all about meteorology. Often they didn't know if it was raining outside the studio or blazing hot. What the producers knew was that these girls had terrific bodies that were very pleasing to the male viewer, and the TV studios put them in scanty lil' costumes. All they were able to do was to read what was handed them and point to a chart that had the area temperatures printed on them. The object was to get the viewers to watch their station by whatever means possible.

Oh sure, it worked great....Guys would miss an address by the nation's president but not the news. That practice faded away and was replaced by trained people who would not only tell what the weather was for the past few days but could also tell you why it was what it was. When the space program was first begun one of the arguments for the huge expense was that weather could be predicted weeks in advance. Not so, oh anemometer breath....They can't predict any better now than they ever could. Don't mess with Mother Nature....She's still the boss and shows us that she is every once in awhile. Luckily we have never been without weather as far as I know...so far.

November 16, 1994

DUCT TAPE
...the miracle of

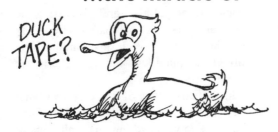

Geez!...Was there a life before duct tape? It's been a long time since any product has become so widely used...it hasn't quite caught up with baling wire but it has taken over some of the chores that baling wire used to have. Check it out, there are cars driving around with whole windows knocked out of 'em and until they can get the glass replaced, a piece of plastic held in place with good ol' duct tape will serve the purpose.

This winter I have lost count of how many nylon or dacron coats and jackets I have noticed that are patched with that trusty aluminum colored fabric tape..."don't stand too close to the stove, Jake, you'll burn a hole in yore coat."..."Aw it's okay maw, I've got a bran new roll of duct tape out in the shop."

Rubber boots that get holes in 'em from crawlin' through wire fences are easily patched up with duct tape and I've lost my addition figures on how many tennis shoes that are existing only by the sheer might of duct tape, the only thing that is holding the body and sole together, orrrr is it canvas and rubber?

Check out the hitch hikers along the big highways like I-5...if their clothes aren't held together with duct tape, their suitcase is. The darn stuff will stick to almost everything that needs patching or mending.

They use it by the mile around TV studios and sound stages for sticking down electric cords and cables to concrete or wood...also keeps people from tripping over the loose wires.

A lot of the small privately owned airplanes (and maybe some of the big ones) use a lot of duct tape..seal off drafts in the cockpit, close up tears in the fabric where a rock or foot may have punched through the covering, aaand it was only a few years ago that some clown changed the numbers on a stolen airplane by utilizing the wonders of duct tape...quick change, now you see a G and now you see a C or a 7 becomes a 1 in the blink of an eye.

The stuff is found on parcel post packages, water hoses are patched with it, blower pipe joints are held to each other with it and I hear they even use it to seal up around a vent pipe or a cooling vent or heating vent...wait a second, isn't that what it was originally made for?

Baling wire is still the more versatile of the two I guess, for a couple of reasons. Baling wire is reusable again and again and duct tape isn't. Baling wire will stand a lot of heat like when you have to tie up a loose exhaust pipe. On the other hand, duct tape won't rust or tear your shirt or scratch up your hands. I guess both products have made a place for themselves in this life of ours and we have come to rely on both of them to get through our daily routines.

Hold the pliers Jake, he won't need 'em...he's usin' duct tape.

February 22, 1989

RUMINATIONS

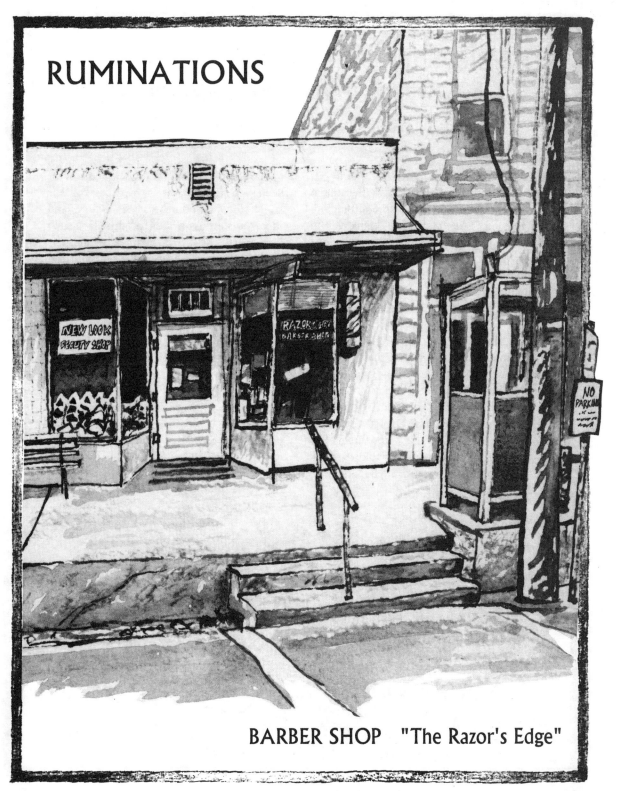

BARBER SHOP   "The Razor's Edge"

THE BIG WIN

P. T. Barnum was right, "there's one born every minute"

Y'know, I've reached a point of complete indifference as to whether or not I will ever win one of these confounded, dingbusted, dadblamed, blank and blankety blank giant sweepstakes that flood the postal system. Not that I ever really expected to win the bigee, like the whole enchilada of 12 million or so, but a couple of times I thought I might be getting close to one of the smaller prizes...like $1.95 or sumpthin'.

I think if I would win something over one million I would just be breaking even, taking into account all the postage I've used sending back those entry forms. I guess it was Reader's Digest that first roped me into this sweepstakes thing. I've been sending those return envelopes back to them for over 25 years, maybe longer.

Here lately every Tom, Dick and Hector seems to be running a sweepstakes for something, and they're getting more and more boisterous in their promises of each and every one of us being a winner...of something, not necessarily the big top drawer prize, but something.

I know you have all gotten these big envelopes with gaudy colors that shout at you, "You may have already won one of our big cash awards"....It does sort of get a person's attention though, doesn't it?

I think I'm at the point when I would appreciate a little honesty from the promoters of these sweepstakes things. F'rinstance, it would be very refreshing to get a big envelope from one of these outfits, say Publisher's Clearing House, that said, "Sorry pal, you are a loser. Don't

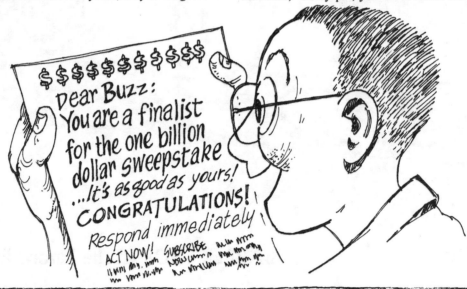

even waste a stamp sending this junk back. You haven't got a chance." Like a cool breeze on a summer afternoon, real earthy honesty.

Ed McMahon and Dick Clark always say, "You may see us driving up to your door to announce that you have won our sweepstakes." For a few years I thought every time I saw dust from a vehicle coming down our road that it might be ol' Dick or Ed. Nope, it was always somebody else, like the PP&L truck coming to read the meter or some guy looking for a lost cow or horse.

Wouldn't it be better to get a big envelope from Reader's Digest that had printed on it, "You missed winning by a mile, not even close. We cannot believe how far off you were in the final drawing."

How about the ones that say, "You are only one in 900 people in Etna to receive this opportunity to enter the final round of our giant sweepstakes." I think those are pretty good odds, considering there are only about 800 people in Etna. Evidently those folks in Pleasanton, New York, don't get into Etna too often.

In the meantime I'll be waiting for that big chunk of mail with the good ol' straight shooter message on the outside that says boldly, "You lost sucker...but you lost big." Or one that says something like, "Go on fool...send in the forms, but you haven't got even the slightest chance of winning anything." Yep, I am definitely finished with all sweepstakes and lotteries...no more!

See who that is commin' down the road....Is it a big gray haired guy with a younger fella that looks like a pile of hair with a face under it?...Is it, is it "THEM?"

October 12, 1994

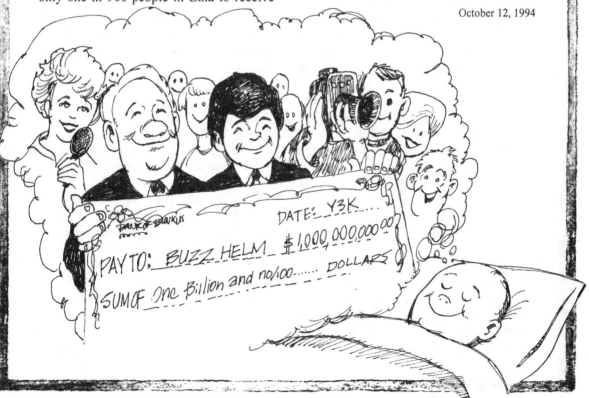

BUZZ PONDERS ON OLD SAYINGS

And 'tis remarkable that they
talk most who have least to say.
Mathew Prior (1664-1721)

Y'know, it sure is funny how we humanoids get hung up on the patent phrases isn't it. I'm sure you understand what I mean.

F'rinstance, anytime somebody asks, "How are you?" we automatically reply, "Fine." I even catch myself doing that in the doctor's office. I'm sittin' there on that cold stainless steel table with a temperature of 103 degrees, and the doctor walks in and asks, "Well, how are you?" I groan out, "Fine, doc, jes' fine." What makes a fella do that anyhow?

Every once in awhile we hear a new one though, and that makes up for all the old trite, antiquated ones like when there's an opening for an affirmative answer to a question. We've all heard, "Do the bears sleep in the woods?"...(I had to alter that one a bit), or, "Is the Pope Catholic?"

The other day I heard, "Do McDonald's counter girls have pimples" I almost came unwrapped at that one. It was new.

It's the same way with a negative answer. We've heard, "No way!" a lot, or "Fergit it!" and "In your dreams." Last week I heard a fresh one. This guy replied, "Highly improbable ol' chap." I think he was some kind of foreigner or sumpthin'.

It's best not to put too much faith in some the old adages of yesteryear. I found out about one when I was a real tender age. It was "Early to bed, early to rise, makes a man healthy, wealthy, and wise." Bah! Humbug! Rubbish, I say.

I tried that when I was about ten years old. It wasn't hard to do 'cause we lived on a ranch or farm. When the chickens went to roost, I hit the sack. When the rooster crowed in the morning, I got up. This went on for about three weeks and nuthin' happened, I had no money, I was dumb as a post, I caught a head cold, and I also had my tonsils out during that time.

"Waste not, want not." I can remember that line from the movie about Lizzy Borden, the lil' gal who put the ax to her parents. Her dad said that at the dinner table one evening when the cook showed him a pot of lamb stew with lil' wriggly things in it. He said, "Heat it up, Dracilla, waste not, want not!" Maybe the ax treatment was truly justifiable homicide after all.

"If wishes were horses, beggars would ride." Sure, I guess so if all you had to say was, "I wish I had a horse." and there, all of a sudden appeared a horse. Or, "I wish I had a watermelon." and plunk! There's a big ol' ripe striper sittin' there. That one I can understand.

I don't really think there are any new ones replacing those old ones, so we can be grateful for one small favor anyhow.

In the meantime, keep your chin up, your back straight, walk a true line, and keep your eyes on the sky....You'll step in a hole and hurt yourself pretty bad.

June 24, 1998

...ponders and ponders and ponders and.....

Where in the world do you suppose some of thuse old sayings got their start? D'ya know what I mean? F'rinstance..."It fits me like a glove." Whoever said that for the first time must get his gloves from a different source than I have.

I get mine from Harbor Freight and fit is accidental, if at all. I don't know who makes 'em for good ol' Harbor Freight, but they seem to think that all the digits on a hand are equal because all the fingers (including the thumb) are the same length on these lil' articles of work apparel, but the price is right.

"Everything is just hunky-dory," orrr, "Everything is Jake..I have never been able to make any sense out of either one of these....How do some of these things get to be a part of our conversation anyhow?

"That just suits me to a tee"....If that old saying is referring to the way a tee shirt fits, it's not very satisfactory...or else I'm not the right build to wear tee shirts.

"Fit as a fiddle" is another one that I have trouble making any sense out of. I have seen and heard, and I'm sure you have too, some fiddles that were anything but fit...warped neck, loose pegs and glued seams coming apart.

Now, if the saying was "fit as a violin" it might make more sense because I've been told that the difference between the term fiddle and violin was that a violin is a much more refined instrument and having a finer tone etc. I wonder if it has anything to do with the person playing it, whether it's a fiddle of violin.

"Slept like a log" has a confusing meaning. Did the person roll around all night? Did he sleep in with a deck of other people? Did he bark all night? Whazzit mean?

"All is fair in love and war"....Now, if that were true then we wouldn't have all those rules governing those two subjects, would we?

"It's and ill wind that blows no good'....I haven't the slightest idea what that one is all about.

Here's a couple that do make good sense...."Waste not, want not" is an easy one to diagnose, and, "Let sleeping dogs lie" Makes a lot of good sense....He may just wake up grouchy enough to gnaw a fillet off the calf of your leg.

"Don't borrow trouble" is one that goes right along with "Neither a borrower nor lender be"....If you borrow it you're gonna have to pay it back, and if you lend it, you're surely gonna get it back...with dividends.

"Clean as a hounds tooth" is an old saying....So how come we have to get all these shots and everything when a hound bites us. The doc says it's to kill all those germs and stop infection....Oooohkay.

"Neat as a pin," "in the pink," "comfortable as an old shoe," "smart as a whip" and so on....There must be a million of 'em.

It's gettin' kind of late, so I'll leave you with this appropriate one...."Late to bed, early to rise, makes a fella doze off while hauling a big load of hay from Scott Valley to Crescent City." End of quote.

September 18, 1996

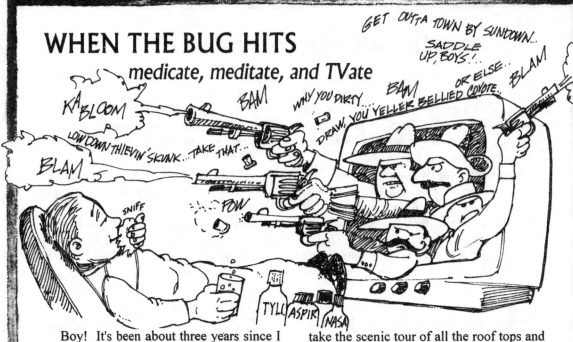

WHEN THE BUG HITS
medicate, meditate, and TVate

Boy! It's been about three years since I have had any kind of bug that has kept me home from work, but this one grabbed me good and put me on the penicillin and Tylox trail for about a week. The Tylox was for pain and it blurred my vision so I couldn't read, but I could see TV, soooo I watched an awful lot of old movies, mostly westerns.

I don't like soap operas or game shows so that narrowed it down to old movies and I thought it might be fun to compare how close to one another some of these old " Oaters" or "Horse Operas" are.

Some of the happening are just alike, no matter if it's a big MGM production or a lil 'ol Republic or RKO effort.

F'rinstance...so often out in back of the bunk house a fella can draw his six shooter and blaze away at a rock or a can and keep it bouncing, never missing a shot, but when he gets into a gun scrape with a "Black Hat" they shoot at each other all afternoon and nobody gets hit...but they do take the scenic tour of all the roof tops and livery stables while they're firing their "60 shooters." Another scenario that's done often...the bad guy has been getting chased all over south Texas, been shot at all day and has shot back all day when finally, finally, he runs out of bullets, click, click...soooo he throws the empty gun at the pursuer. Imagine that, he just throws the gun away. I guess he thought they came loaded and when they were empty you had to go buy a new one. Most of the time he's wearing a gun belt with about 50 bullets in it, and yet...he just throws the gun away and they resort to fisticuffs until one of them gets shoved into the horse trough, then he's done for sure, off to the hoosegow for you, bad guy.

On the other hand, how about this one? A gunslinger has ridden his pony to death out on the desert, or the hoss steps in a hole and breaks his leg, ya gotta shoot him...but wait, what's he doing? The rider takes off the saddle and all his trappings, slings the whole load over his shoulder and heads off into the blazing desert. He won't put an empty gun back in the holster, but he's gonna carry a heavy saddle clear across New Mexico looking for a refill...walks into the first livery stable, throws down the saddle and says "fill her up!"

The old stuff about a lone rider out on the desert in the blazing sun, takes the last swig from his canteen, bone dry, so what does he do? He throws the darn canteen as far out in the desert as he can, juuust throws it away! What if he stumbles onto a nice cool clear spring about nightfall, he won't have anything to carry water in for the next day or two that it will take him to cross that dry piece of trail.

The smart ones always had an Indian pal, Indians always knew where the water was...they were so sure of themselves they didn't even carry canteens...follow that Indian.

Well, thanks to Tylox (the pain pills) I made it through the week of old movies about the early west, but you know sumpthin? I wouldn't turn down a chance to watch another one tomorrow, even if I've seen it before.

November 27, 1985

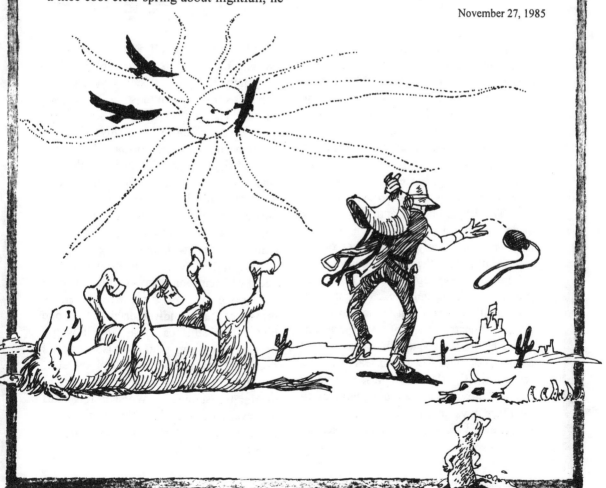

THE BIG SELL

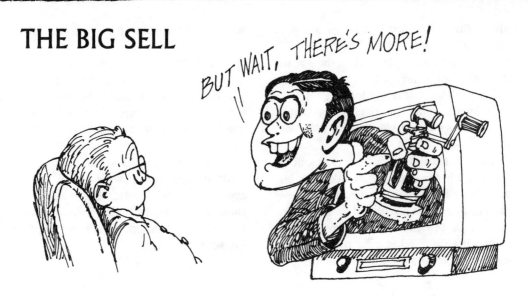

BUT WAIT, THERE'S MORE!

As a rule of thumb I guess we Americans are a pretty gullible bunch of humanoids, and that's a lucky thing for the advertising business....Check out the unbelievable stuff that's offered for sale in magazines, newspapers and TV.

Everybody has some kind of snake oil to cure hair loss, bunions, psoriasis, oily skin, diet to lose weight, diet to gain weight, exercise machines to use up extra energy, etc. The list is endless and these people make healthy deposits in their favorite bank each and every day whether or not their product does the job it's supposed to.

I am sure no exception to the rule when it comes to being gullible... I'm game for just about any scam that comes down the pike. Fortunately, none of my experiences have been the kind that have cost money...not since I was ten tears old and sent for the Charles Atlas muscle building course that would make me the envy of all the other guys on the beach...and no bully would ever kick sand in my face a second time.

I don't have to tell you that it didn't work....One look is testimony to that. Spending money on attractive ads like that one is a very good and lasting lesson....It's easy to just say, "No thank you sir."

I am one of those lucky guys who has never been allergic to poison oak. I have worked right in the thick of it, inhaled the smoke from a fire that was burning it and all that stuff...I've never had the stuff. However, I was told that the resistance could change at any time, and I may contact the rash without warning.

This fella I knew was brewing up a batch of "manzanita tea"...gallons of it. It was only good if it was made from the new growth of leaves and you drink at least one pint of the stuff each day and it would prevent you from getting poison oak. I drank about one thimble full of the stuff and thought, "that will have to take care of me for the summer"....Worst tasting stuff that ever passed my lips, but he said it was good for me, so I took it. Not good for "white eyes," I decided.

A few years ago I started wearing a copper bracelet because it's said to relieve the aches and pains of arthritis. I couldn't tell any difference after a couple of years, so I quit wearing it. I have somehow become older and achier and painier since then and have started wearing the thing again...was it the bracelet? Or the added years? Why take a chance, wear the cotton pickin' bracelet.

I'm proud to say that I passed up one offer that sounded very good but involved money. A fella in Nevada was running an ad offering dry water wells for sale. The deal was, the dry shafts could be bucked up into two foot lengths and sold for fence post holes...no digging, just install the holes in the ground. Sound strange? I'll bet he sold a few.

After all, every year some poor soul buys a state highway bridge from somebody with the idea of making a toll crossing out of it, aaaand look at all the successful sweepstakes gimmicks that are going on....Sure, of course I keep sending them in.

March 13, 1996

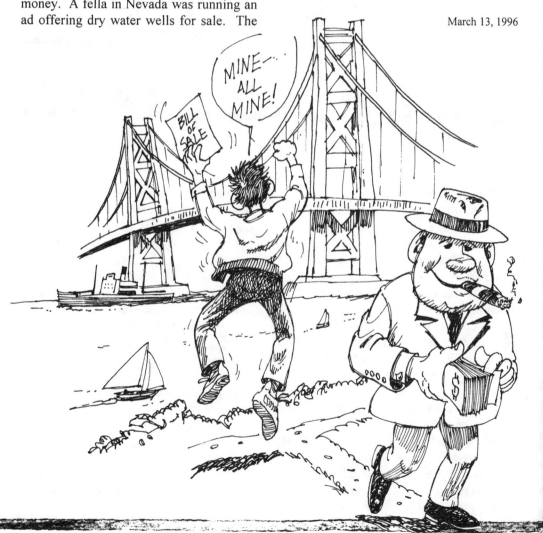

49

(un)TRUTH IN ADVERTISING

A short course in understanding advertising copy.

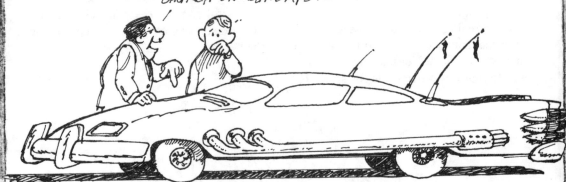

"Let the buyer beware." is a phrase we've heard all our lives, I guess. That's the one that has been changed to "Consumer Awareness" (nothing stays the same) and there are a whole bunch of committees and panels who draw big wages to see that the public is not getting cheated or short-changed.

Of course, we somehow overlook the fact that we are getting short-changed in what these panels and committees are doing to earn their tax-supported paycheck.

Just recently there was a report made public on how used car brokers, as a common practice, roll back the odometer on a used car, make it seem that the car has hardly been driven at all. Sure, it's against the law, but what isn't?

Good, honest used car dealers who buy from these used car brokers are not the ones who pull these illegal tricks, it's the people they buy their cars from who are the culprits.

It was even shown on the TV report how they roll back the little numbers...the only tool needed is a wire coat hanger bent into a little hook and you can set the ol' mileage to anything you like.

I thought it might be useful to have a glossary of terms that are seen most often in relation to used cars that are advertised for sale.

F'rinstance..."This little beauty needs a good home." Probably needs a home 'cause the junk yard was full at the time.

"Low mileage" we just covered, but it also may mean that it has just a tad under a hundred thousand on the ol' carcass.

This one we've seen or heard all our lives, "Owned by a little old lady who only drove it to church on Sundays." They forgot to say that her nephew ran the thing on pure nitro the other six days of the week, just blowing the doors off from dawn to dusk, and in between.

"Needs brakes"...this means that if it would have had brakes it wouldn't have hit the horse and wouldn't be for sale in the first place.

"Good rubber"...the radiator hoses are fairly new.

"Good paint"...uh-huh, what there is left of it.

"Needs tune-up"...right after new rings and a valve job are completed.

When the ad stresses "good upholstery" it may mean that is all that's good about it.

"One owner vehicle"...the poor guy never did have any luck trying to sell that ol' lemon.

Then the champion slogan of them all..."Mechanics special"...look out! These usually have to be towed home and have all (or almost all) of the engine components in the trunk, like a sort of do-it-yourself kit...without the kit.

That same old nagging question keeps chewing away on the back of the neck when you shop for a used car, "If this heap is so good, how come the last guy got rid of it?"

May 9, 1984

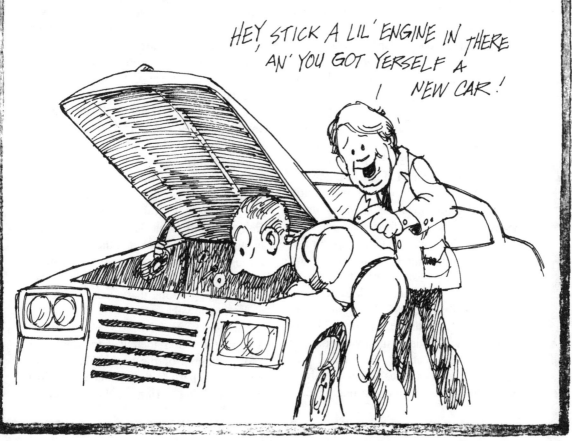

THOSE IRRESISTIBLE REAL ESTATE ADS

The old art of making the silk purse from the sow's ear.

The fine art of decoding real estate ads.

Have you ever heard the story about the fellow who listed his house and property for sale with a realty firm and when he saw the ad in the paper describing his place he liked it so much that he decided to keep it cause it was just what he was looking for?

There is a definite art to writing a real estate ad to make the property sound attractive to the reader, but experience will tell you to read between the lines, over the adjectives, and behind the patent phrases.

Take for instance some of these little gems...."Walking distance to shopping"... means you better take food for three days and a sleeping bag. "Good exposure"... means the bathroom wall fell out. "Secluded"...the last people to see the place was the Lewis and Clark Expedition. "Gentle to rolling hills"...like going from the Swiss Alps to the Matterhorn. "Partly level"...the west side of the living room, if you put a Sears catalog under one leg of the table. "Lots of trees"...pines ready to fall on the roof in one more strong wind.

"Builder says finish it yourself"...means the foundation is almost complete, owner quit when he discovered one side was three feet higher than the other and didn't meet with the ends. "Will build to suit"...buyer gets to choose from three sets of plans that were cut out of an old Popular Mechanics magazine. "Will consider trade"...owner will do almost anything to get rid of this lousy hunk of rock slide.

"Restorable"...you get a set of 1857 house plans and a pile of thick and thin, worm eaten sugar pine lumber. "Close to schools"...means you are only 12 miles from Bill and Edna Schools, your closest neighbor. "Fixer-upper"...the roof caved in last fall and it sat open all winter. "Handyman special"...a certifiable basket case, nothing wrong that a can of gasoline and a match won't cure.

"Seasonal stream"...every March brings a torrential flood then it's dry the other eleven months of the year. "Promise of gold on property"...the former owner lost her wedding ring while picking blackberries one day and never found it. "Undisturbed natural setting"...the place is built right smack on top of a two hundred year old rattlesnake den.

"View of Mount Shasta"...for two weeks in February when there is no fog and before the oaks leaf out in the spring. "Room for a horse"...if you don't mind keeping Ol' Paint in the spare bedroom. "Power and phone are available"...sure, utilities are available anywhere, all you have to do is pay to have the poles put in and the wire strung for about thirty miles. "Lots of fruit trees"...several chokecherry

and mulberry trees and an apricot that hasn't produced fruit since Moby Dick was a minnow.

Even ads for rentals are tricky, here are a couple of time tested terms..."House pets okay"...means the place already smells like a rabbit hutch anyhow. "Small children okay"...the place is beyond repair so why worry. "First and last month's rent with cleaning deposit payable in advance"...owner says, now I gotcha, pilgrim!

June 23, 1982

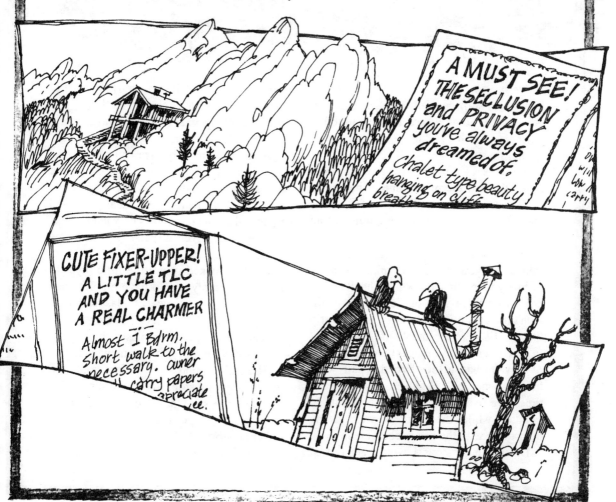

A MYSTERY
...here's the parts, where's the car?

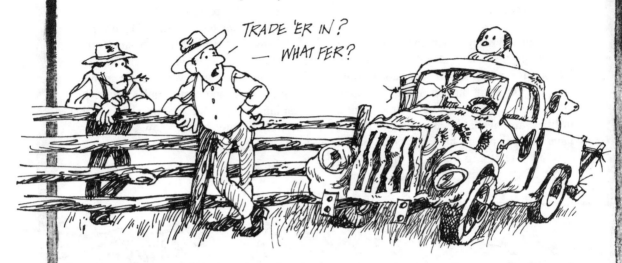

TRADE 'ER IN?
— WHAT FER?

I've been wondering for a long time just how much stuff can fall off a car before it gets to the point where it can't function anymore...ranch pickups are an even greater mystery.

It seems like every city parking lot I have ever had the misfortune of having to use is seasoned with all sorts of lil' parts that, at one time, were the trappings of an automobile.

Small bolts and nuts, tiny springs, rubber gadgets and cotter pins, once in awhile you might see a whole shock absorber laying there with one end broken off. Don't the cars miss this stuff? On one trip that the ELW (ever lovin' wife) and I took to Las Vegas (Lost Wages) the great state of Nevada had a lot of road repair work being done on Highway 395...several times we were stopped for at least 20 minutes while the workers were doing their thing with the heavy equipment.

During these stops I would get out of the car and stroll up and down the highway near the car, sometimes just strolling along gazing at the gravel along the shoulder of the road.

Amazing what you see...hub caps, gas caps, oil dip sticks, even saw one whole fender once. A hood or two out in the brush, wiper blades, the usual nuts and bolts and I can't remember how many caps, gloves (but never a pair), shoes (same thing), jackets etc.

If I had picked up all the little mystery items I probably would have a coffee can full in no time...pieces of plastic, metal, chrome and rubber. bits of red or yellow reflector type glass or plastic pieces are always there in the gravel somewhere.

The ELW found a pretty darn good pair of pliers at one stop, they were just laying there in the sand near some sage brush. Now, ranch type pickups are a whole different story.

They lose big pieces of stuff, not on the

highway, but in the fields and around the scatter. Stuff like a whole tail gate or a head light...once in awhile an oil pan or a radiator...but they notice that usually.

I've opened bales of hay and found fan belts, one glove and stuff like that. Once there was a sleeve from a denim jacket in a bale....I was a little hesitant to dig further in that one, could be an arm in there, but there wasn't.

You can study a ranch pickup for a few minutes and come up with quite a long list of stuff that is noticeably missing...like doors and windshields, tailgates and

fenders etc., but, on a passenger car that spends most of it's life on the highways, it's hard to find just where those little bolts and nuts, springs, rubber washers and cotter pins fell from.

Eventually enough little items fall off to cause a problem I suppose, but there's never a warning before it happens. Maybe that's why those ranch dogs are always barking when they ride in the back of the pickup on a trip to town...they're hollerin', "Hey Boss!..sumpthin' jest fell off the rig."

July 12, 1989

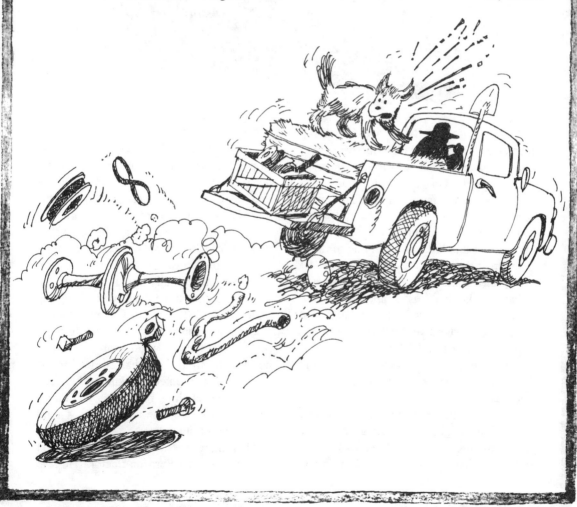

OF MULES AND MACHINERY
which is the more intelligent?

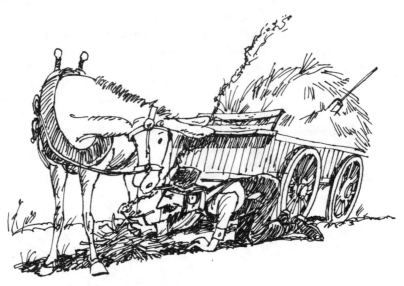

Y'know, looking back and rerunning memories from growing up days, I'm convinced that machinery is just as smart as an animal. I'm gonna talk about farm machinery and farm animals...by your leave.

I remember as a kid they used to tell a story about this fella who had one of those stubborn type mules. Most of the time he was pretty good about doin' his work and behavin' like he was supposed to, but every once in awhile he would just rebel...wouldn't move or budge from his stand. His owner didn't hold with whippin' or beatin' one of his animals, so he would just wait till the critter decided to move and then he went.

He loaned the mule to a neighbor one time....The neighbor had an ailing horse and needed to get some old straw cleaned out of the barn so he borrowed the mule.

He got a pretty hefty load on the wagon and got out of the barn with it okay. He stopped to open a gate to the field where he was takin' the straw, and when he swatted the mule to get going again the mule balked...would not move an inch.

The fella decided it was time to break that ornery beast of his bad habit. He took some of the straw and built a small fire under the mule's belly, not a big blaze, but some uncomfortable heat was rising up under the mule's carcass. The mule looked back for a second and then moved forward just enough for the wagon load of straw to be over the lil' fire and balked dead in his tracks. He seemed to know the fella would unhitch him before he got burnt, which he did, but the wagon was a total loss. That's thinkin'!

Then there was this guy who owned an old iron wheeled Fordson tractor. He also owned one of the hottest tempers in the county...quick and hot. That ol' tractor would quit on him once in awhile way out in the middle of 60 acres...just stall and wouldn't start.

The fella would take out his big ball-peen hammer and start workin' that tractor over...poundin' on the wheels, radiator, hitch, hood, or any part within his reach and then walk to the house and phone the mechanic from town to come and fix it.

He finally had the tractor so beat up it just wasn't worth repairin' and the mechanic told him so...and suggested he buy a new tractor.

The farmer gave in and bought a brand new Farmall...red one with rubber tires and a padded seat cushion. Well, Sir/Mam, that darned new fangled tractor stalled on him way out in the middle of nowhere, and he just couldn't get it goin' again....Up came the temper and out came the hammer. He busted the lights, pounded in the hood, caved in the radiator grille.

His last act must have been takin' a big healthy swing on one of those rubber tires because just about dark, late in the evening, they went lookin' for him, and there he was...flat on his back, hammer in hand, and a big knot on his forehead the size of a goose egg, right between the runnin' lights. His lights were out for a couple of days...concussion or sumpthin' like that.

One for the machine, zero for the hot tempered farmer....That's thinkin'.

October 25, 1995

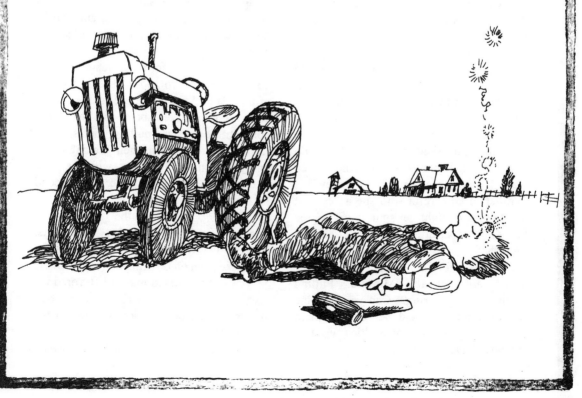

MARLAHAN MUSTARD CAPITAL OF THE WORLD? ...*making the most of it*

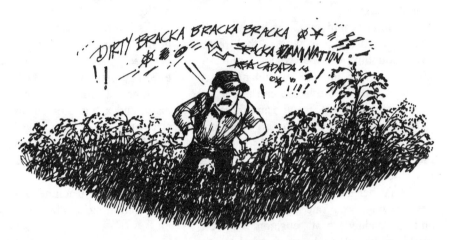

Y'know, I've mentioned this idea before, but I didn't press hard...just tossed the idea out to see if it would fly. It didn't....It just crashed and burned with deafening silence.

With partial jest I'll make another go for it. The subject is mustard weed, or as the tourists call it, that beautiful yellow flower that grows so freely amidst the alfalfa and wheat fields.

I can remember a lady from Santfrunsisko asked me once, "What do you call that pretty yellow blossomed plant that is so prevalent in the valley?" I told her to be careful who she asked that question, she might get some third degree burns on her ear drums...not Bayarea-type English.

Anyhow, forging ahead here....How about an annual "Mustard Pulling Festival" every spring? Can you imagine two or three thousand people out there crisscrossing the valley, pulling up this noxious single rooted plant.

The stuff isn't hard to get rid of if everybody would fight it. In the cool days of spring while the soil is moist the root comes right out of the ground and can be done before the blooms mature and spread more seeds.

The idea of forming teams for a combined effort to add a little zest to the affair....We Americans are supposed to enjoy competitive sports so why not competitive mustard pulling contests. The teams would weigh in their "catch" at the end of the day. The team with the most plants would win first prize, then second prize and finally third prize.

Think of the spin-off possibilities...bumper stickers, tee-shirts, mellow yellow balloons, mustard puller caps, key chains. Maybe even Uncle Steve's old fashioned mustard flavored ice cream, or the Etna Brewery's mustard flavored bock beer...a definite first in the grog world.

We would, of course, have to have a

Mustard Queen Contest for each and every year. The contestants would all wear mustard yellow bathing suits and the winner would be driven around the valley in a mustard yellow 1956 Chevy pickup...after the Mustard Pulling Festival Parade, of course.

Lest we forget, horseradish put Tulelake on the map with their annual Horseradish Festival....Crescent City has it's crab races, Carson City has their camel races, and Angel's Camp has the frog jumping contest....People don't think they are stupid festivals...dumb maybe, but not stupid.

The big annual event could culminate with a good ol' Mustard Puller's Ball where the winners of all would be the valley agricultural community by eliminating that weed.

It would maybe even become so endangered that it would have to be planted each year just to accommodate the annual Mustard Puller's Festival. What's that? It's a stupid idea? Oh, okay...never mind.

April 29, 1996

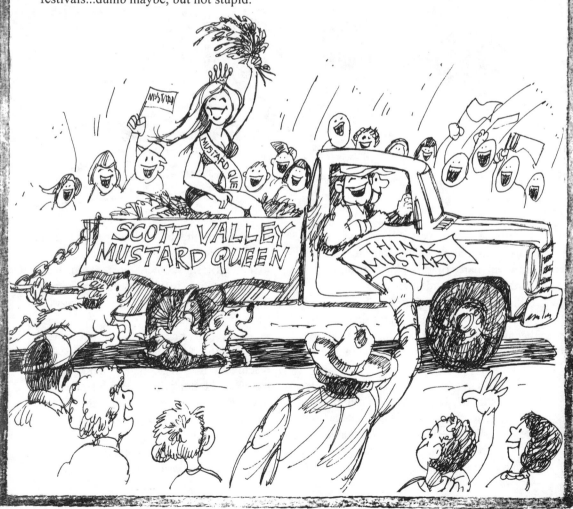

59

ON EATING
not for the squeamish

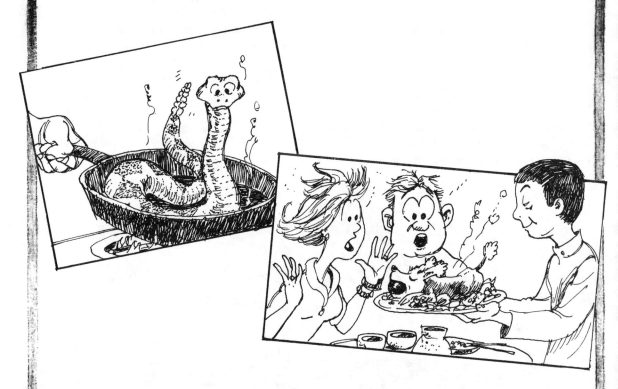

You are what you eat!...Aww, geez, I hope not. Eating habits that are found in different parts of this planet that we call earth are varied and interesting.

The National Geographic Society tells us that in some remote parts of the world cannibalism is still practiced, so you gotta be careful how you accept a dinner invitation.

"Would you like to come over for dinner this evening? We had one of your missionaries for dinner last night, he was delicious!" Ah, err, ummm, no thank you, I gave up missionaries for lent, orr some dumb excuse like that.

I was talking to a fella from Esquida, Old Mexico, who told me he dearly loved to eat rattlesnake meat, just couldn't get enough of the stuff, went out and hunted the things all the time. Fried 'em with hot salsa and jallapenos.

I said that I never had eaten rattlesnake meat but that I had been told that it sort of resembled frog legs in taste and texture. He said, "I don't know Senior, I would never in my life eat a stinking frog."...Oh, ahhh, I see.

Reader's Digest reported on a couple who were touring China and they had their lil' pet Poodle with them...never left the thing home. It was not only a dear pet to them it was one of the family. They went into this Chinese restaurant and as usual the dog was with them on a leash and they led him to the table with them when they were seated.

They ordered their meal as best they could with the non-English speaking waiter and then wanted to order something for the Poodle so he could dine with them. After much difficulty with words and sign language and to the Poodle and making eating motions, the waiter finally got this big grin on his face, he finally understood.

He took the Poodle and disappeared into the kitchen. After waiting for over an hour, the waiter come to the table and put this big silver tray in the middle and removed the big oval lid...lo and behold there was the lil' Poodle with an apple in his mouth, roasted to a tee.

The lady keeled over in a faint and the man went to the authorities who explained that it was not uncommon in that part of China for customers of restaurants to bring in a small pig, a dog a cat, etc., and ask the kitchen to prepare it for them. Sorry, no case for the courts, round eyes.

One time my uncle was invited to a big outdoor Basque celebration out in western Merced County near a town called Dos Palos. They had these big caldrons on open fires with great juicy things cooking in them that smelled terrific.

Uncle Les bounced the ladle on the bottom and dished up some strange looking and good smelling items, one of which resembled a water chestnut with somewhat the same texture...yum-yum.

He asked one of the sheep ranchers there what that thing was, he was gonna get another one with the next helping of stew. The big Basque fella said, "Ah, haahh, Leslee! You are one luckee man, that is the eye of the sheep!"

Uncle Les said, a few days later after he had recovered, that the guys who got sheep's eye from the stew pot were supposed to have real good luck all year long.

That's not really so bad...have you ever gone through a baloney factory here in this country? If you like baloney don't take the tour...a word to the wise.

April 5, 1989

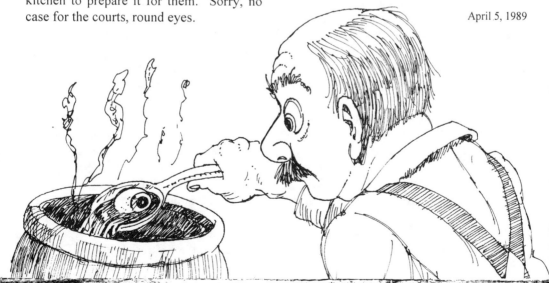

TRAVELIN' AND EATIN'
a word to the wise....beware!

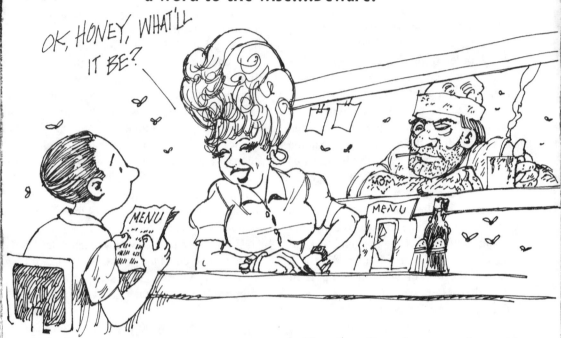

OK, HONEY, WHAT'LL IT BE?

MENU

MENU

A few years ago, a country western singer by the name of Ray Stevens, made a recording of a song about how he hated to get a haircut on the road and away from home and he went on to describe some of the experiences he had in some of those away from home barber shops and how some of them weren't really barber shops at all...just beauticians pretending to be barbers and cutting men's hair.

Ever since I heard that record I have often thought how I have had some awful experiences in cafes and restaurants on the road and away from home. Now, I don't mean on the big concrete ribbons like I-5, those eating places are mostly chain outfits or franchises and, although they may not be great, they are uniform and you pretty well know what the food will be like.

The places I'm going to mention are the little joints on the little out-of-way hamlets on those two lane highways that meander all over the state to get you somewhere...you know the ptomaine taverns I mean, they most often have a really neat, well planned sign out in front of the place that blares out with all the softness of an air horn on a Kenworth truck.

Tricky worded signs with letters eight feet tall that say, "EATS"...real classy, and underneath a smaller sign that says, 'Pets Welcome"...? The cooks in these places all look alike, dirty t-shirt, toothpick behind the ear and a cup of black coffee on the edge of the grill and usually about a day and a half away from a shave.

Him and the waitress are usually mad at

each other about something or other. These guys have one unique talent in common, they have the uncanny abiliity to be able to cook an egg with the yolk hard as a rock and the white is left runny...??

Heaven help you if send something back to the kitchen for a re-do...you won't recognize the junk when it comes back to the table and is slam dunked in front of you on the ol' worn and faded formica table top.

In one of these places one time I heard one of the customers order the, "specialty of the house." When the waitress finally got to our table I asked her what the "specialty of the house" was and she said it was hash so I told her I'd try the hash and she hollered to the cook, "We got another daredevil here, Red!"...??

It wasn't all that bad, as hash goes, but the coffee was the worst I ever tasted in all my life...terrible! I heard the waitress ask a guy at the table next to us if wanted a refill on the coffee and he replied in a loud voice, "I'd rather be horse whipped than drink another cup of that stuff!"

Some guy on the other side of the room said, "If I'd known there was a choice I would have taken the whip right at the start." The waitresses in these places must have all gone to the same polytechnic school of gum snapping...smack, smack, smack, pop, smack, etc, etc. "D'ya want somethin' else?....Tums? Rolaids? Alka Seltzer?" Snap, smack, pop...Naw, just gimme the check...by the way, how can I get to the nearest freeway from here.

November 1, 1989

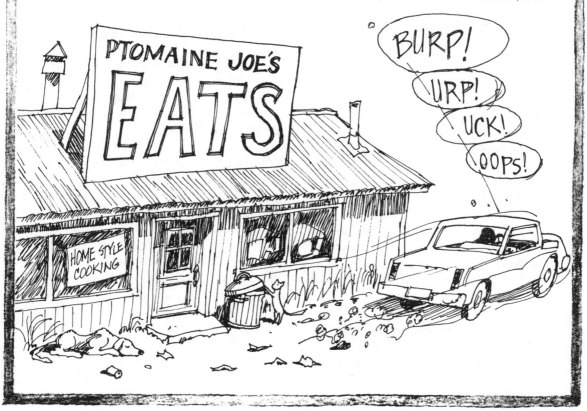

MORE TRAVELIN' AND EATIN'

Y'know, I've found out something about being on the road alone. The restaurants would rather have single customers sit at the counter. They're not really happy with having one person taking up a whole booth. The person that sits the customers will invariably say, "We have seats at the counter."

See, these are things that I have to get used to. Traveling alone that is. If at all possible I won't sit at the counter again if I can avoid it and I'm gonna explain why.

Not long ago I took a trip down south to visit relatives and I got hungry somewhere down there along the way and pulled off the freeway and went into one of the chain restaurants that are noticeable from the road. The hostess informed me there were seats at the counter and I told her I would really rather have a booth. I told her I was a big tipper. She said, "And I'm a Dallas Cowboys cheerleader. Besides, all our booths are full." Okay, I sat at the counter.

It's hard to find something to look at when you're at the counter, you either look in the mirrors behind the counter or you watch the cooks in the kitchen. While glancing in the mirror I noticed that the fella next to me kept staring at me; just a steady level stare. I finally asked him, "Do I know you?" He never even blinked and he asked me, "Did you know the earth was flat?" I told him I had heard some talk about it, but most people think it's round. He said, "Oh, it's round alright. Like a Ritz cracker. It's round but it's flat." I told him that was a theory they didn't discuss when I went to school. He continued,

"Yep, if you drive on a straight line long enough you'll drop right off the edge. Zoom! Round like a pool ball." The waitress brought my sandwich and rolled her eyes as she sat it down. I got the idea that she knew all about this guy and felt a little sorry for me being seated next to him.

The fella continued, "An I'll tell ya' about sumpthin' else. Y'know all that malarkey about goin' to the moon? Well, that whole thing was done by a Hollywood film studio right out on the Nevada desert, yessir!" I began to get a little worried because by the time I got to my potato salad, this guy was beginning to make sense. Dangerous stuff, and I was eating way too fast because I just wanted outta there.

The waitress brought my check and as I was downing the last drop of water from my glass this fella says, "Say, did I hear you mention that you were headed for Sacramento? I'm lookin' for a ride south."

I lied right through my teeth and said, "I'm sorry, did I say Sackamenna? I meant Seattle. that's north y'know." The waitress was rollin' eyes again. It sorta made me feel bad that I had told a fib, but if I had that fella's company all the way to the edge of the world I might become completely unwrapped and do something very bad. Next time I'm gonna say, "Please young lady, could I have a booth? Even one in the rest room is okay, anything but the counter.

December 16, 1998

JOY OF CUTTING THE CHRISTMAS TREE
fun, fun, fun, in the great outdoors

Here are your 1989 guidelines and rules and regulations for cutting your own Christmas tree. The very first thing that you must do is to obtain a permit....Go to your local forestry headquarters and pick up one permit for each tree you want to cut, they're only two bucks apiece. They will give you a nicely printed sheet of instructions on how to stay legal on the tree hunt and cut.

Plan your trip well ahead of time. Above all, don't go while the weather is decent, that takes all the adventure out of it. Pick a day when the wind is so strong it's tearing the manzanita out by the roots and is about one degree below "too cold." When the big day arrives check your equipment before departing...have the signed permit with you, take a saw or small ax, have a CB with channel nine capabilities, splints of various sizes, a tourniquet or two, red or orange emergency smoke flares, dress warmly and leave a copy of your last will and testament with someone you trust.

Never, repeat, never put on tire chains until your pickup has slid off the road at least three times or has become completely unable to be moved in the direction you wish to go. Of course, while getting the chains out, you all of a sudden remember you never did get around to repairing that broken one from last season, (plenty of time...got all summer) so, of course, that must be done under the worst conditions.

Never cut the first tree you find, even though it's the most perfect one you've ever seen. It's just not done old chap, you must search, walk, hike and change your mind at least 20 times before you go back to that one you passed up at the start of the safari. For the utmost of enjoyment it's imperative that you drop your ax or saw at least once during the trip, in a place where it will slide a long way down into a gully or ravine. After retrieving it and finally arriving at the tree that was selected you discover that there are absolutely no limbs on two sides of the poor thing.

Finally, after the wind has increased considerably and the temperature has dropped another ten degrees with the snowfall getting heavier, a tree has been selected and amputated at the ankles, placed in the pickup and headed for home. By the time you get home your hands should be thawed enough so that you can make a fist and the circulation has improved in the rest of the body to enable you to unload the prized quarry...another successful Christmas Tree cutting sortie has come to an end.

No matter how homely that lil' tree may be when you are dragging it out of the pickup, it's always the prettiest one you ever had after it's in the cave and decorated out in it's finery...."Honey, this is the best one we ever did have!"...."I know it sweets, and hardly any trouble at all!"

November 29, 1989

I SHOULD HAVE KNOWN

...the agony thereof

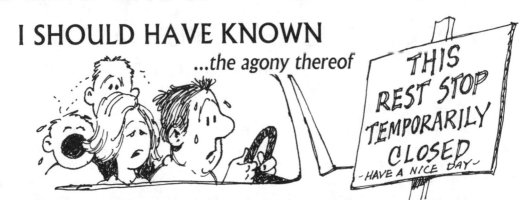

There are some little minor inconveniences that happen in a person's life that can be expected but not counted on...although more often than not, when they happen, we say to ourselves, "I should have known."

Take f'rinstance this little scenario...you've been driving on a long stretch of highway and it's been a long time between towns and you get so thirsty that you feel like a camel herder on the ninth day of a ten day trip across the Sahara, when all of a sudden you see this sign, "Rest Stop, one mile ahead." The first sign you see when you pull in is a hastily scribbled bit of information that says, "Sorry, closed temporarily, no water"...dad blast the ding busted, I should have known.

Perhaps on a trip out of town you get a motel room and get all settled in, figure you'll catch the late news on the TV...uh-huh, just as sure as taxes, the darn TV doesn't work....I should have known.

How about the times you use a public rest room and wash your hands, reach for a paper towel and there aren't any, so there you are with dripping hands ...handkerchief time.

Maybe you've driven around a large parking lot looking for a spot to put the ol' heap in and you finally see a vacant space about three rows over...when you get there it's got a motorcycle sitting there that wasn't visible from a distance. Or, how about this one, you've had a real hectic week with meetings every night that lasted till ten or eleven o'clock and you finally get a night when you have nothing to do so you crawl into the easy chair to read a little bit before hitting the hay, when here comes company and you can bet the first thing they will say is: "Fer gosh sakes, in your pajamas already? You must go to bed with the chickens." or words to that effect...grrr. I should have known.

Have you ever planned and looked forward to a camping trip up to one of the lakes? Maybe you've planned the trip for a month...you get there and one guy says to the other one, "Heck no, I thought you brought the eggs." It doesn't matter to much, the other fella forgot the frying pan anyhow.

Oh well, just sit back under that big fir tree and enjoy the three days of rain, without eggs or pancakes..."Naw, I thought you brought the coffee." ...I should have known, doggone it!

June 26, 1985

PARSLEY...AND OTHER IRRITATIONS

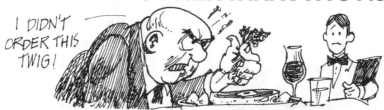

I DIDN'T ORDER THIS TWIG!

There is probably a real good reason for a lot of things that seem to not make any sense. Come to think of it, maybe it isn't a good reason at all...maybe it's just some dumb law that makes the management of businesses do these things.

Take for instance (f'rinstance) parsley. Now, I don't know about folks, but I don't choose a restaurant by the quality of their parsley that is always tucked away someplace on the dinner plate. Did you ever hear anyone say, "Let's go to Fignewton's Cafe for dinner tonight, they serve the best parsley."...?

I don't think that I know one person who rushes through his prime rib in order to casually enjoy his sprig of parsley that's peeking out from under the baked potato or the spiced apple slice. Oh sure, it's a handy item to twirl between the thumb and forefinger during idle conversation, but there's been darn few times that I can remember actually eating the little green morsel.

Have you ever seen a TV commercial where some cranky little ol' lady yells, "Hey, where's the parsley?"

I figure that parsley growers of America have a real strong lobby and have forced legislation to force food people to include their product on all dinner order. I'm just grateful the 'possum growers are not that well organized. Sometimes when I'm in a real weird mood I'm tempted to ask the waitress if I can substitute star thistle for the parsley, but she would think I was nuts asking for star thistle when it's out of season.

Another thing is, in hotels and motels they have this little strip of paper across the seat in the bathroom that proudly states "Sanitized for your protection." How is that little strip of paper going to protect anyone from anything? And how do we know they didn't do a real hasty job of cleaning the room, like just changing the sheets, putting up fresh towels and gluing that strip of paper across the throne lid?

Maybe it would be a good idea to pack a can of spray Lysol with us when we travel and do our own sanitizing...but with so many agencies looking out for our protection, that's probably not really necessary.

After all, on the parking deck there are signs that say to lock your car for your protection, and in the room on the door there is a little sign that tells you to use the night lock for your protection and if that is not enough, a person can always take a little paper strip from the bathroom and stick it across the door just for added protection...and maybe stick a sprig of parsley in the keyhole...it's gotta be good for something.

May 16, 1984

IT WAS A DARK AND STORMY NIGHT

rule number one: stay indoors!

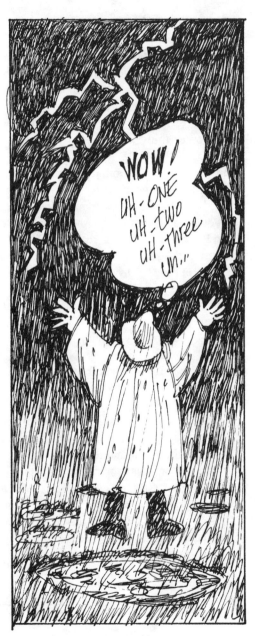

Just off hand, I can't think of anything as refreshing as a good ol' thunder storm at the end of a long dry hot spell. That one we had the other evening was just great, lot's of rain that even had some moisture in it. Plenty of bright lightning in the sky. I know, I know, lightning starts fires but, as long as we can't do anything to make the lightning stop we might as well enjoy the phenomenon.

Statistics say we, that is each and every one of us, stand one chance in two and a half million of ever getting struck by lightning...about the same chances of winning anything in the lottery I guess.

They (whoever "they" are) also say that we have 50 times more of a chance of being drowned in some sort of water accident than having a bolt of lightning hit us.

I came across a couple of formulas for measuring how far away the lightning is from where you are standing at the time it flashes. One goes like this...count the seconds from the time you see the flash until you hear the thunder clap then divide by five. That will give you the distance in miles.

If it's really close, you can do the same thing only instead of dividing the seconds by five, you multiply by one thousand...this will give you the distance in feet that you are from the strike.

If it's real close you can smell a sort of sulfuric odor from the strike. If it hits so close that you can taste it...that is a sensation of taste in your mouth that might liken to chewing on a galvanized nail, you are too darn close, move away a bit. If you see the flash but no smell or taste is noticeable, don't worry about it...your relatives will handle all the details, make all the arrangements.

A fatalist, they tell me, is a fella who thinks that if it's meant to be that he gets smacked by lightning, then so be it. A optimist thinks that he is the one person that will never ever be struck by lightning.

A pessimist is a guy who thinks that if anybody will be hit by a bolt of lightning on that day, it will be him. Wellll, I don't know about those outlooks on things. They used to tell me that there were two ways of looking at the misfortune of loosing a button off your shirt...a pessimist thinks he has lost a button but an optimist thinks he has gained a button hole. Just like one fella thinks his cup is half empty and the other thinks it's half full...to me it all seems to work the same.

I try to make it a habit to stay indoors during an electric storm, no point in tempting fate I always say, that is, sometimes I say that...actually, I can't remember the last time I said that.

Fortunately, a storm that lets go with a lot of lightning is not so bad if it's followed by a good heavy rain...that helps snuff some of the "hot" strikes that may have started a fire up in the woods.

I wonder if there shouldn't be some sort of federal funding to send a crew up in the timber to soothe the poor spotted owls who (hooooty-hooo) may have become overwrought at the threat of being struck in the tail feathers by a hunk of lightning...sort of "feather strokers" or some such title.

August 16, 1989

GEEZ, I DON'T KNOW. THE LAST THING I REMEMBER, I WAS STANDING THERE COUNTING THE SECONDS FROM THE LIGHTNING FLASH, AND THEN....

ON KEEPING WARM
there is real heat and there is make-believe heat

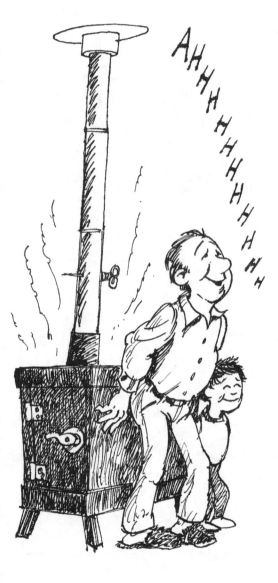

With the almost perfect weather that we've had this fall, it's hard to get very interested in preparing for the winter that is bound and determined to happen. One of the up front things to think about in winter preparation is some method of staying warm...that's important.

A lot of folks still rely on that good ol' wood heat. I don't know about you folks but it's very important to me that I have a wood stove in the house...I just have to have something to back up to when I come in from a harsh, freezing winter day. Central heat systems are okay I guess, but where is the main epicenter of heat to warm up the ol' hip pockets? We have an assortment of methods of heating our big ol' century plus aged house...electricity in some parts of it, a fancy computer operated oil furnace in another part and wood heat to back up everything else in case the is a failure of either power or oil delivery.

We could survive on any one of the three heat systems but I would miss the wood heat the most. How much wood does the average household need for the winter you ask? Welllll, that depends on a host of factors...how big is your teepee, how cold a winter, what kind of wood you are burning, how much are you home and how warm do you like to keep the ol' cave.

There is one dependable rule of thumb...too much wood is just perfect. Some guys watch the squirrels and judge the severity of the coming winter that way.

F'rinstance, the more acorns and nuts the squirrels are gathering, the longer and colder the winter is supposed to be. On the other hand maybe the squirrels are watching the humans...the more wood the humans haul in, the more nuts the lil' squirrels gather up, thinking the humans know something they don't about how bad the winter will be.

I don't want to alarm anyone or shock them back into reality but...there are only about 68 more days until Christmas (fiendish grin and impish leer) and prices are already on the rise for the "Season of Good Will and Fellowship."

The ol' mail box is stuffed with special Christmas catalogs already. I think most season type shoppers are prone to buy nice cozy warm things as gifts for the adult world...warm fuzzy slippers, thick cozy sweaters, fluffy jackets with fur collars, a scarf and ear muffs etc.

These are the things that are priced for the season...why not buy summer stuff, those things should be priced to move quickly and they sure would be appreciated next summer. Just think, brand new summer stuff to unwrap the first of June, just like a second Christmas in the year. Of course, there would be some disappointed faces around the tree on the big morning...unwrapping a new swim suit when you were expecting skis.

About three or four times a day I get asked, "Well Buzz, what kind of a winter are we gonna have this year?" Now, I know these folks trust me to give honest, straight-forward information, so without hesitation, I look them right square in the eye and answer, "I'll tell you on May 30, 1990 about the winter season."

I know they appreciate my honesty cause some of the guys signify that they think I'm number one...by holding up one finger.

October 18,1989

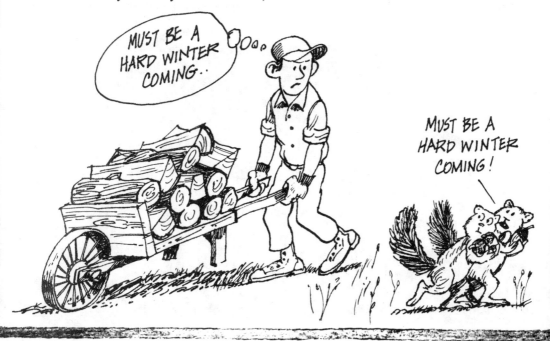

MUST BE A HARD WINTER COMING..

MUST BE A HARD WINTER COMING!

EL NIÑO ~ LA NIÑA
who cares, snow is snow

There's an old saying that we have all heard plenty of times that says, "Too much wood is just enough," and that could probably work just as well if you said it about hay too.

Most people usually plan on enough wood to last them through the winter. They figure about how many cords it takes to warm the ol' teepee from the fall of the year 'til spring.

There's just something about the word "Spring" that seems to warm up the blood and makes us think that when spring gets here we will all at once have to start squinting our eyes against the sun and shed one layer of clothing.

According to the calendar, that magic time of the year is supposed to hit on the 21st of March and some little malfunction, in a human being's working parts, nudges us and says, "Well, that's it, we made it through another winter." Well, pilgrims, just a little reminder about that springtime business and some of our false intuitions that can lead us astray.

There've been a lot of years around these parts when the only difference between winter and spring was the time of the day that the sun went down. Springtime can catch a fella with the woodshed empty and about twenty inches of snow all around the scatter and you find yourself trying to decide whether to chop up some seldom used furniture for firewood or spend the day pushing a shopping cart around the inside of a nice

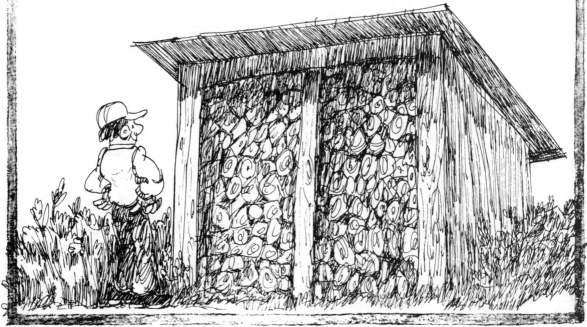

warm grocery store, trying to look like you're shopping, so nobody will guess you're just in there to stay warm.

Most years it's too darn wet and muddy to go out and cut any wood in the spring. If you try it, you might have to wait until August to go back and get your pickup where it was left, up to the tail lights in mud.

It's also pretty scary when you find yourself gettin' pretty far back in the barn fetching hay. One day you pull off a bale and there's the boards on the back of the barn staring at you and you think, "M'gawd! it's either spring or somebody shortened up the barn. And if it's spring, how come there's so darn much snow on the ground."

Well, fortunately it's not the end of the world; there are people around who have learned a thing or two about the seasons and they are very happy to sell a few cords of wood to tide you over, orrr a few tons of hay to get you by for awhile.

Maybe the summer is the real cause of our shortsighted idea of how much wood we need. When a fella is all tired, hot and sweaty from bringing in a load of wood and chucking it in the shed, it's real easy to think, "Shucks...that'll be about enough to get us through 'til spring."

Everybody knows that this idea of cutting firewood for two or three winters ahead of time is not logical...just plain not logical.

March 2, 1983

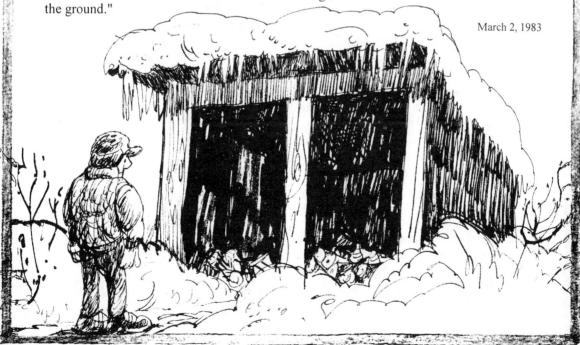

WINTER DRIVING?
...forget it!

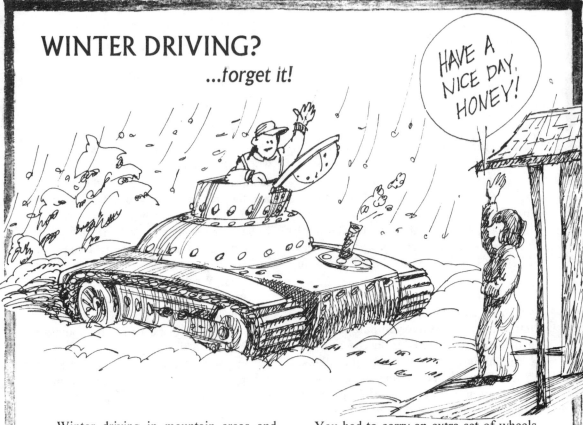

Winter driving in mountain areas and how to cope.

Number one rule of thumb is if you don't own a WW-2 Sherman tank with steel tracks...stay at home. If you have to travel in stormy weather or freezing conditions there are a couple of things to remember, like, carry tire chains with you aaand take along some hardy individual to install them for you if the need arises.

Over the years there have been many innovations to make winter mountain driving easier and safer. One of the first things other than chains that I can remember was a tire that was recapped with rubber impregnated with walnut shells, they were great on snow and ice but lasted about as long as a bowl of pretzels at a beer festival on dry or bare pavement.

You had to carry an extra set of wheels with the walnut tires mounted on them so you could switch back and forth. Later on different types of so-called "traction tires" were made available, some had steel shavings from lathe machine cuttings in the rubber instead of nut shells and they became a fire hazard...steady stream of sparks when they hit dry pavement...kinda like chains.

The steam railroad engines that the McCloud River Lumber Company used to run in the winter had sand hoppers mounted on them with a spout that emptied right in front of the big driver wheels... gave them great traction.

The big freight truck companies took this idea and put the system on their big trucks for icy road conditions and more than once I've followed one of those rigs over icy mountain roads and stayed in his tracks to scavenge on the sand trail he was leaving...worked pretty good usually until the trucker decided to pull over and take an hour or two shut eye.

Traction devices have improved over the years with lighter material of some of the new plastics but they still haven't come up with a way to put them on without getting outside in the weather to do it. The fella that comes up with a way to install chains from the inside of the car and stay nice and warm and dry and cozy while doing it will become independently wealthy in just one winter.

A good snow tread tire with studs installed is about the best thing going for icy snow at this point in time but they are not the perfect answer either. F'rinstance, have you ever been behind some car when one of those steel studs came loose and hit your car like a bullet? It's exciting alright.

If you are unable to locate a surplus Army M-32 medium tank with steel cleats that you can buy, orrr a good ol' half track with a big Diamond-T engine in it, then I would suggest a list of things to have with you in your car if you just simply have to get on the road during those icy snowy conditions.

Of course you should have your traction devices (chains, etc) and a good reliable flashlight, gloves, insulated waterproof coveralls, hard hat, sheet of plastic to lie on, pliers and bailing wire for repairs to chains, Band-Aids for repair to fingers and hands and a nice selection of wooden clothes pins...to put on your lips so you can't open your mouth to scream out all those nasty, dirty cuss words.

Happy motoring, Pilgrims.

January 18, 1989

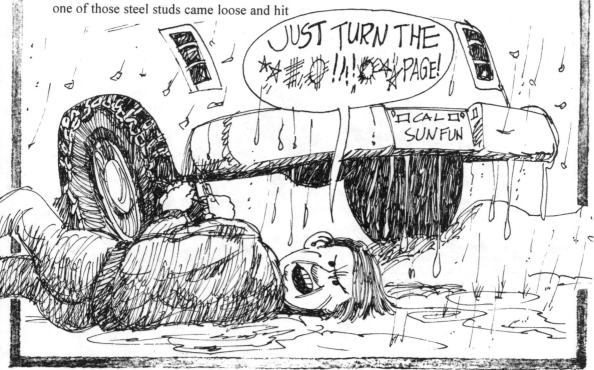

FAVORITE HOLIDAYS
Christmas 1 - Groundhog Day 0

I guess I have to say that Christmas is my favorite holiday and has always been my favorite. Perhaps mainly because of what it symbolizes and the history of it. I'm sort of a holiday nut...I like Thanksgiving very much and rate it right up there next to Christmas. I like Bunker Hill Day a lot too, and rank it right up there near Thanksgiving. The Fourth of July is a great one too, and I rate it right up there next to Bunker Hill Day. Easter is a really nice holiday and the symbolism is a real tug at the heart strings. Ground Hog Day is terrific also and I rank it right up there next to root canal work ...

One of the things about Christmas as a holiday is the smells, the aromas, the odors that the ol' nose picks up that are distinctly associated with Christmas....Know what I mean? F'rinstance, the smell you catch when going into stores, scented candles, fresh spruce, fresh fir etc. The house parties...boy, the house parties! When you first walk into the host's house you get these smells of hot cider and cinnamon sticks...spice candles burning and the Christmas Tree sending out it's aroma.

Around our scatter, the ELW (ever lovin' wife) goes into her cookie baking frenzy every year just about two weeks

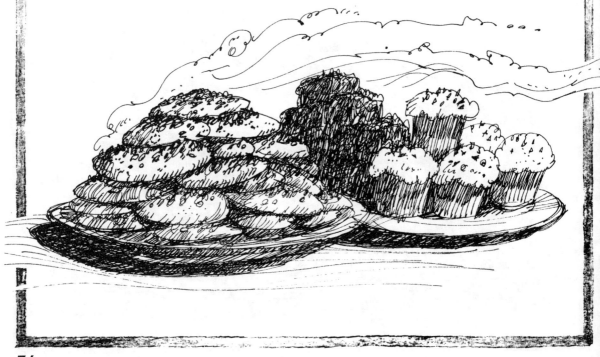

before Christmas. Five different kinds of cookies and about six dozen of each kind. The oven goes constantly until the deed is done. The aroma sent out of that kitchen is enough to cause the average guy to gain five pounds of weight just from the air in there.

There's one recipe that she has for a super tasting cookie called "Christmas Rocks"....Wow! They'll blow your doors off. They have to sit overnight after the dough is mixed ...covered tightly to seal in all the goodness. How the smell gets out of that big tub of dough with the sealed cover over it I'll never know, but the aroma seeps out. I swear sometimes I can hear the ingredients in that big tub gurgling and sizzling when I walk by....It's just throbbing to get into that oven and become cookies. Once in awhile I'll snitch a fresh,

out-of-the-oven warm cookie as I walk through the kitchen. That's when I can almost hear and see Dr. Nancy saying, "You've got to watch your weight, Buzzy."...."Shucks Doc Nance, I don't have to do that....You're watching it close enough for both of us."...Yuck-yuck! Oh-oh...not funny.

I guess Ground Hog Day is about the only one that nobody ever cooks a special dinner for. I shudder to think what the main course might be...probably not turkey. Bunker Hill Day is June 17, the date of a big battle during the Revolutionary War, annnnn, it's also the ELW's birthday. See how come we don't cook a big dinner at home?

December 14, 1994

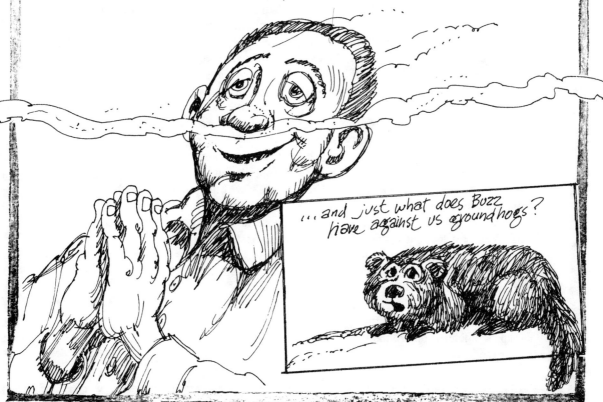

A BLACK AND WHITE CHRISTMAS
...generically speaking

Last week a fella said to me as he was departing..."Let me be the first to wish you a very generic Christmas." It was a good shot and we both had a good chuckle over it, but he was right ...he was the first one that had wished me a generic Christmas.

Now, that little bit of humor got me generic conscious and since then I've been noticing this generic stuff more and more. Seems as though all generic products are packaged with a plain black and white label which makes them stand out on the store shelves real noticeable, like a raisin in the sugar bowl.

They have generic canned goods, generic cigarettes, generic dried foods, generic this and generic that, even generic wines!!...As well as generic vitamins and drugs for prescriptions.

The prices of generic goods are very attractive and I suppose the quality of the merchandise is good, but I sort of believe that most of us are brainwashed into the thinking of most promotional firms. The public goes for attractive packaging, fancy bright colors on the labels and all that stuff. Welll, maybe, but if that's true how come we notice a black and white car on the highway and can detect and confirm that it's a Highway Patrol car out of all the other cars on the freeway, aaand...it's just a bit short of being pleasing to the eye when your speedometer is up around the 70 mile an hour mark.

The more I thought about this "generic Christmas" thing, the more I had visions zipping through the ol' noggin.

Let's try to picture a generic Christmas...a black and white Christmas tree?? A black and white Santa Claus?? With black and white reindeer? Shucks, they'd look like Holsteins. All those presents under the black and white tree wrapped in black and white paper. Black and white lights on the tree and a lot of black and white holly and mistletoe hanging around. I know the real meaning of the Christmas season would certainly be the same, that's constant, but it would not as pleasing to the eye. We'd probably be saying things like, "Well, if you've seen one Christmas tree you've seen 'em all," and stuff like that.

I hasten to say that it's every one's privilege and right to have any kind of a Christmas they want, orrrr...none at all, but from me and the ELW (ever lovin' wife) here's wishing each and every one of you nice folks, a full blown, all color, non-generic Christmas....Hope you have the merriest, brightest, most joyous holiday season ever and may the good Lord take a likin' to ya.

December 18, 1985

REFLECTIONS

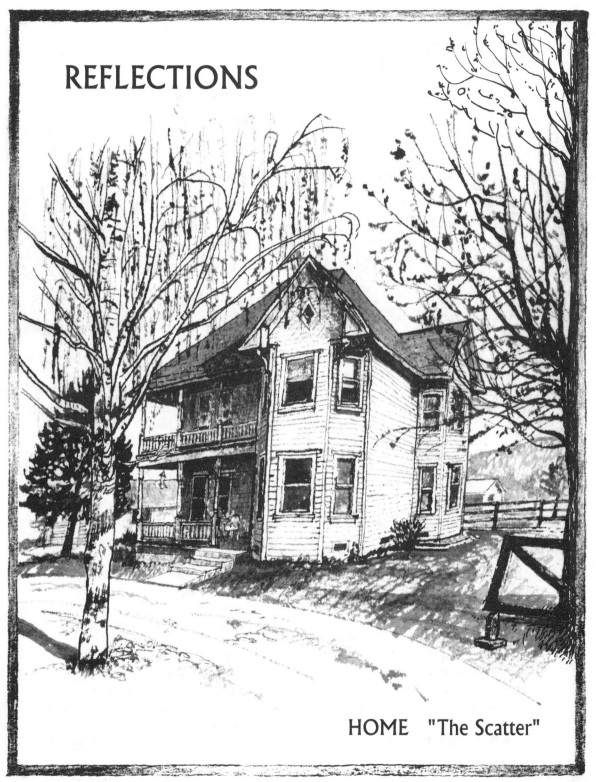

HOME   "The Scatter"

THE OLD SUNDAY DRIVE

*Ahhh, those wonderful days in the back seat; windows down,
head out, watching the world glide by.*

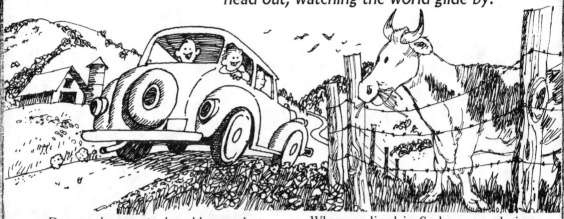

Do you happen to be old enough to remember the "Sunday Drive"...? Y'know what I mean dontcha? The Sundays that Dad would get the old family whoopy out and the whole family would enjoy a drive to some place and come home in time for dinner, orrr if it happened to be a time when the family wallet was in pretty good shape, we would all get to eat out for dinner.

I can still remember the Sunday drive that ended up at a Chinese restaurant on the way home....It was the first time I ever ate at a restaurant. I was awe-struck...and the most memorable thing was that Mom didn't have to clear the table or do the dishes. Fantastic! What would they think of next?

The ELW (ever lovin' wife) and I used to do that Sunday drive thing when our two lil' moppets were in grammar school, and they really did enjoy that outing with all of us together. We ate at restaurants a lot more often than when I was a kid, but that's how things change, I guess.

When we lived in Sackamenna, during our absence from Callahan, we used to take frequent Sunday drives up into the Mother Lode Country...visit the old mining towns and stuff. Most of the time we would pack a picnic lunch and find some secluded, shady spot along the American River to eat and frolic.

When we felt flush enough to eat at a restaurant we had our favorites. F'rinstance, there was an old hotel and restaurant in Sutter Creek that served family style and the food was plentiful and good. It had a 20 foot ceiling in the bar, really high...and the ceiling was covered with business cards that were put up there with thumb tacks.

The first time we went there I asked the guy how in heck he put those cards up there without a ladder, and he said, "Gimme a dollar, and I'll show you." Wellll, okay, I gave him a dollar and he stuck it in the cash drawer and exchanged it for a silver dollar.

He said, "Gimme your card if ya got

one." I gave him my card, and he put a thumbtack through it, laid the silver dollar in the palm of his hand, and put the card on top of it...very deftly tested the wind and the distance, and tossed the dollar and card up. SPLAT!...The dollar came down and the card was tacked to the ceiling. He gave it to me strictly on charge to never reveal the secret of how it was done, lest his little lucrative sideline would become less profitable....Far out!

That was just one of the interesting lil' things that we found out about on those wonderful Sunday drives, and the kids remembered them into their adult lives.

I hasten to inform you that gasoline was about 19½ cents a gallon at that time and staying home watching TV was an unheard of misuse of time during the beautiful summer months.

August 14, 1996

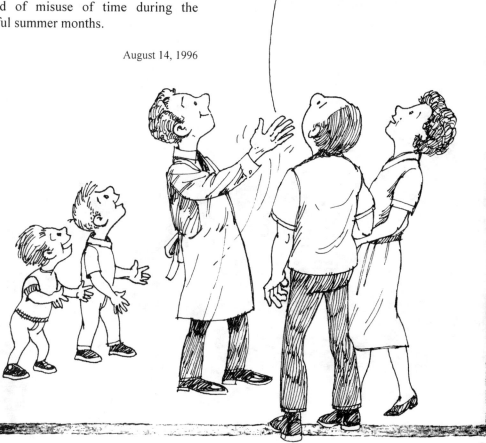

SUMMER GUESTS

It's a migratory thing.

Oh boy...! Summer is here with all the little spin-off times that go with it, like more work and projects than we can ever hope to accomplish before the winter hits us again.

Besides the regular normal repair that stuff always needs and the new things that have to be finished by fall, and firewood to get while we are resting, there is another thing that looms up, a thing that happens to us but is seldom if ever talked about candidly and openly and a thing that we meet with mixed emotions; the situation is...visits from friends and/or relatives who decide to spend a few days of their vacation as house guests up here in the country away from the city, especially from those far away and mysterious places like "Sakamenna," "Lozangeles," "Sanfrunsisko" or "Sanazay."

More often than not it happens around one of the holidays like Memorial Day or Fourth of July...about a week or so before the big weekend a letter or a phone call comes that starts out, "Good news, we have decided to come up and spend a few days with you country cousins"...ohhh, ahhh, gosh, that will be just ahhh, ummm, great, (Dammit...! I was gonna move that fence and fix the barn roof.) sure, come on up, it'll be swell seein' ya.

City people really do mean well and try not to rearrange your life too much while they are visiting...they usually make it clear that they just want to be here and not interfere with the normal activity and flow of events like, they'll offer to help with any projects that you have going on around the diggin's and will come out in the field bright and early (about 10 AM) wearing

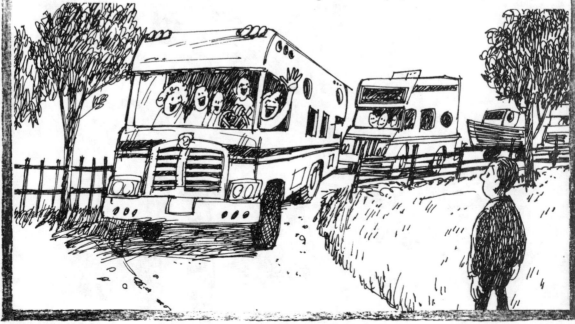

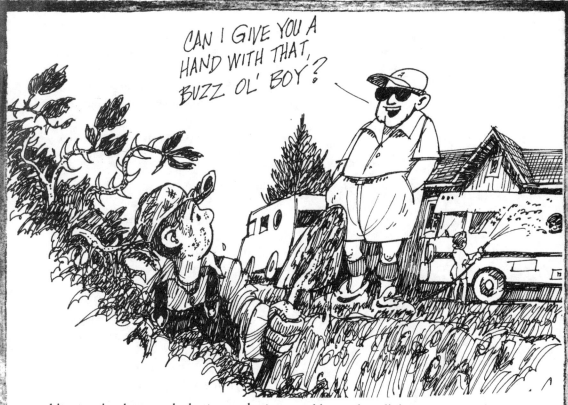

white tennis shoes and shorts, ready to help you tear out that bunch of berry vines and brush along the ditch, offering good advice like, "You ought to run all this water through a big pipe, saves evaporation." or, "Why don't you train these cows to go potty in one place all the time instead of all over the nice meadow?" an "You could hire somebody to do this kind of work and have more spare time."

Sometimes they have a fluffy little dog that spends all his time in the house except to go outside once in awhile and find something dead to roll in and then come right in the house just as proud as he can be...at dinner time. Some of them take 20 baths a day and wash their big motor home or car and camp trailer twice a day ("Well...it's dusty.") and the ol' pump motor on the well gets red hot while PP&L

adds another digit to next month's power bill.

They want to stay up all night and sleep most of the morning away. Finally they pack up and leave and as you watch them going down the road, waving them good-bye, you have to admit to yourself that it sure was nice to have them visit and it was enjoyed after all, but one thing always bothers me...when I go to visit them at their place, how many irritating and annoying things do I bother them with?

I hope for the best and think that maybe it's about even but I'm afraid I may be much worse...at best.

June 2, 1982

OFF TO SEE
THE MOUSE

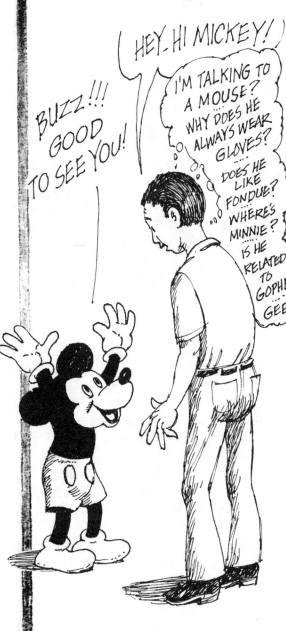

Have we ever discussed the fatefull trip to Disneyland that happened about 1958 or '59? It was the first visit to that wonderful land that dear ol' Walt built for all kids...nine to ninety...orrr younger and older.

The ELW (ever lovin' wife) and I had scrimped and saved to get up enough cash that we could take a week's vacation with the kids, and we decided to surprise them with the trip to Disneyland. We didn't tell 'em until almost the day we left....We were afraid something might happen to cancel out the vacation. We visited Disneyland with the muppets several times, but there's nothing that can compare with that first-time experience.

We had been on the road about an hour when Sheri, the youngest, began her, "Are we almost there yet?" routine....We're talking about 11 hours of summertime through the valley drivin' here....Tempers can rise as well as temperatures. Rick, the other child, wasn't so bad about wanting to get there in a hurry...he always wanted to know how far it was to the next take-out food joint.

I have to say that the Disney Park was more than I hoped....It was just fantastic. We took all the rides once and some two or three times, visited all the shops, and ate an awful lot of food. The ELW tore the seam out of the back of her "peddle pushers" getting on the burro for the Grand Canyon ride...had to tie Rick's sweater around her waist to avoid becoming an added attraction along the trip.

That was the only mishap, but it turned out okay. They sent us over to the costume department where the ladies in there sewed up the tear and made everything right again.

It was a wonderful day's enjoyment, and also enjoyed taking the kids to Hollywood, Grauman's Theatre, the Wax Museum and all the hand and foot prints on the sidewalk. The days went swiftly, and all of a sudden it was time to head home.

The fella who ran the motel said if we wanted to a take real nice and scenic route home, we should take Highway 1...right on the coast all the way, beautiful scenery...ocean view all the way up the coast.

Okay, we did it. We got on Highway 1 at Santa Barbara, hit fog as thick as clam chowder before we ever saw the ocean....It got thicker as we progressed northward.

After a couple of hours I developed that ol' pain in the shoulders and neck...eyes smarting from squinting at the tail lights of of the car ahead....Traffic had slowed to about 20 mph.

Sheri pipes up, "Are we almost home?" and Rick chimed in with, "Dad, I'm hungry. When are we gonna eat?" The ELW says, "I'd like to drive a spell and relieve you, but I just can't handle foggy driving."

All of a sudden there appeared a pull-out area, and there was a great big building that was a combination grocery store, clothing store, gas, cafe and fishing equipment. They were sold out of all food except chili. I have never before or since eaten such incendiary chili. I can sure understand why the store was all sold out of Tums, Rolaids, and Di-Gel.

We finally got into Santa Cruz and I cut over to good ol' hot and dry Highway 99...no fog...just unbearable heat...happily on the last leg of our trip. From the back seat comes, "Are we almost home, Daddy?" and "Are we gonna stop and eat pretty soon, Dad?" Aaaand, "I'd offer to drive Hon but I'm just whipped."

Noooo prob, I'm fine....We gotta do this again sometime, right?

April 17, 1996

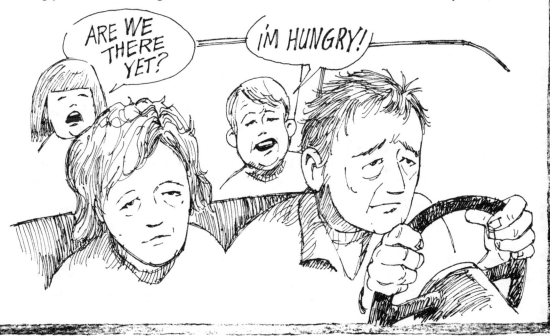

HOW NOT TO TAN

...OUCH

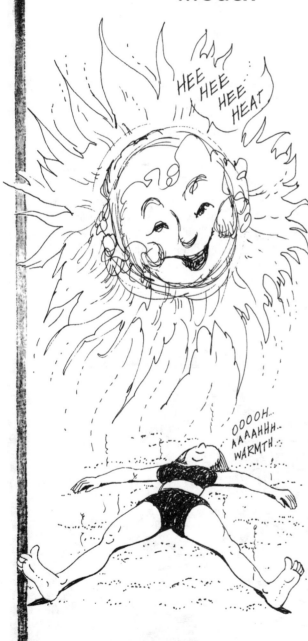

HEE HEE HEE HEAT

OOOOH...
AAAAHHH...
WARMTH

Sunburn!...Oweee! These early summer days the sun has extra super strength in it I think. Some of our young folk have started the summer season early by getting flat top and butch haircuts and the first thing that happens is, their ears and forehead get cooked.

When I was a young kid (yesss, they had sun then) my nose and ears were one solid blister all summer, I could almost watch the tiny lil' bubbles form up and break. My brother and I used to see who could get the largest chunk of peeling skin off in one piece...he always won.

I think it was because he had a bigger body or something, but he would get a piece off the upper arm sometimes that would sound like adhesive tape being ripped off and it would be big enough to cover the palm of the hand...yechh!

When our kids were smaller we used to take our vacations in San Clemente, on the ocean and beach, you know...take in Disneyland and the San Diego Zoo and all that Lozangelus stuff.

We had this favorite motel that was almost on the beach...the "C-Vue Motel" I think it was. It was our favorite because it was the cheapest motel in town...a double bed and two roll-aways for the family for a mere five bucks per day ($5) but you have to remember this was a bunch of years ago and the top price in town was probably $15...see, when you're talking cheap you use the term "bucks" and if it is expensive you say "dollars."

The sand on that beach at San Clemente was almost white as snow and this one year that we were there our skins were as white as the sand on that first day. We had so much fun, it was the first time we tried riding the big ones in to shore on an air mattress...if we didn't have movie films as evidence I would never believe I had done anything like that.

Anyhow, as the day wore on we all began to get redder and redder, but the ELW (ever lovin' wife) took the prize for the most vivid crimson.

That evening we all trooped into the local drugstore downtown, it had big signs in the window that advertised a stuff that would take the pain out of a sunburn. Somehow the kids and I were the first ones in the door of the store, the ELW was having a lil' trouble getting the back of her knees to flex so she was walking slower than the rest of us.

The guy in the store said, "Whoooaah! You guys have some kind of sunburns there." and was in the process of fetching some stuff that would ease the suffering. About this time the ELW comes struggling through the door and the guy's eyes almost popped out and he said, "Holy Toledo! Wow! Hey Orville, come out here and take a look at this one, you won't believe it!"

Orville came out of the stockroom and goes through his amazement routine and mentions how he has been living on the beach all his life and never before saw a walking barbecue like that one.

He gave her some stuff that he said was used for the after burn of the atomic bomb at the test site in New Mexico and chuckled,...a real comedian. The other fella said, "Don't let daylight touch you for three days, even if your room catches fire, don't go out in the sunshine." Not one of our most pleasant vacations, but one of our most memorable.

April 26, 1989

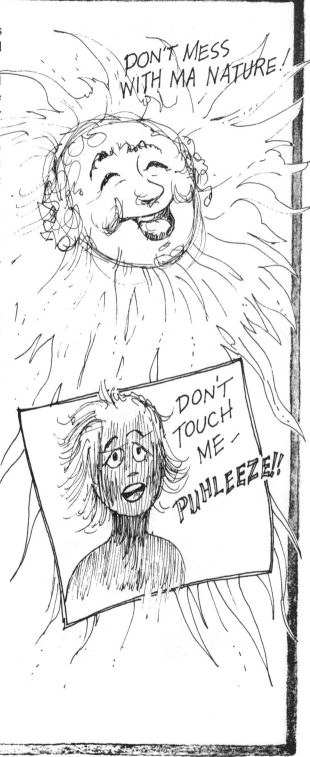

SCHOOL DAZE
memories, sweet and sour

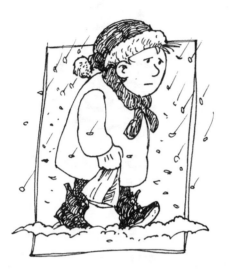

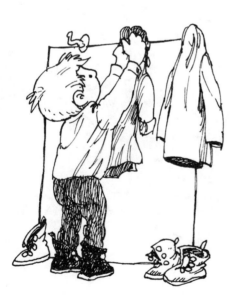

Well, school is going full blast again. Just about one hundred percent of the young folks agree that the summer just went zipping by...the teachers mostly agree with the young folks...that it was a short vacation from school. Seems to me that everything goes ripping by at a fast clip....I can still remember some of those first days back to grammar school like it was just yesterday (well, almost) and some of my early impressions of things in those days.

The second and third grades in particular stuck to my memory, especially the third grade...I did that one twice. I think they just held me back to give the teacher a hand with the new recruits that year..Another opinion was that I had my name on the "dunce cap" more than anybody else...they should have made me a present of that thing when I finally passed the third grade, it was almost beginning to shape my head, I had to wear it so much.

The first day back in school after a summer off was sort of fun. You got to see a lot of the kids that you hadn't seen since school let out for vacation.

In our school we had a long narrow room at one end of the classroom that we called the "cloak room" and that's where you parked your "stuff"...we all had "stuff" then.

You know...lunch buckets or dinner pails as some kids called them. I always had a brown paper sack, that's what most of the farm kids had. The town kids had regular tin pails that held their lunch neatly without mashing the bread and banana together with the roast beef and berry pie. You had to save that paper sack and use it all week...and the waxed paper, too. After lunch we'd fold up our little paper sacks and tuck 'em in our back pocket to take home for a refill the next day. Every Monday you started out with a brand new paper bag. Way in the back of my mind I had this fear that if I lost that paper bag, or threw it away mistake, I wouldn't get a lunch again until the next Monday, orrr, that I would have to stuff my lunch in my pockets for the rest of the week.

In the winter time the cloak room was full of coats and sweaters and golashes (overshoes) and everything had to be neat...coats hung up on hooks, lunches on the shelf and overshoes (golashes) near the heater to dry.

The cloak room always had this heavy odor of Rose Hair Oil mixed with the smell of oranges, apples and bananas. The classroom itself had the odor of pencil shavings and chalk dust. The teacher was always a lady teacher and looked about 80 years old to us...actually she was probably around 35 years old. She knew everything and could see everything that was going on, even when her back was turned. She had this uncanny knowledge of who was not paying attention too...that's when she would say to you those words that struck sheer terror..."Go to the board and write what I just said." That would always do me in, I could never remember anything she said after, "We will now stand and pledge allegiance to the flag." That was way back at the beginning of the day...right after an hour on the bus, when we were still alert...sort of.

August 28, 1985

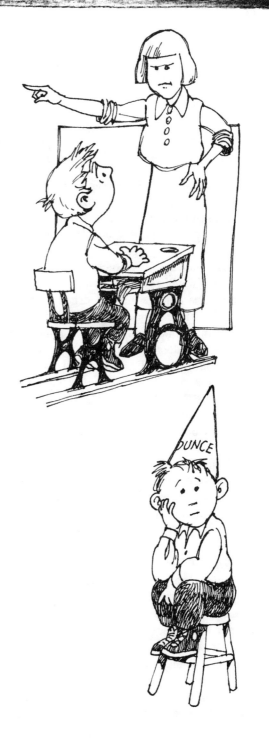

I'MAGONNA'S
...and all those other big plans

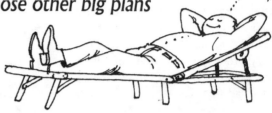

I'MAGONNA—.... TOMORROW.... I THINK... MAYBE.... ZZZ

This is the time of the year when we can sorta reflect on all the "I'magonna's" that were so carefully planned back there in the spring...you know what an "I'magonna" is ...this summer I'magonna clean out that willow patch along the ditch.

One of my big priorities was to fix some sort of a barrier over my woodshed door to keep the rain and snow from dripping right down my collar when I'm opening or closing the door. Just some sort of an overhang was all I had in mind, with a kind of a gutter to run the water some other direction than swishing straight off that tin at about ninety miles per hour.

Under ordinary circumstances I can shut that door and hook the latch with no problem, but when it's raining it's a very time consuming and complicated matter and takes forever...transposing time to water flow, it sometimes takes a good two and a half gallons down the neck to get that simple task done.

When it's not raining or snowing, it's a flat one and a half seconds, tops. The rain is pretty uncomfortable, but the snow can be a lot more of a surprise. F'rinstance, after a heavy snow there might be as much as four or five inches of the white stuff on that old roof...then along comes a day when there is a little bit of sunshine and it begins to loosen up and slide off...pretty often the time it picks is when I'm hassling that latch or maybe just that little vibration from slamming the door closed is enough to shake it loose.

Anyway, when that big section of snow hits a guy on top of the head and covers up an armload of wood it doesn't make fumbling with that latch any easier.

By golly, that reminds me. Next summer I'magonna change that door so that it opens in, instead of swinging out then it won't be barricaded by snow drifts ...an' that's another I'magonna that will probably turn into an "Iwuzgonna".

What's an "Iwuzgonna" you may ask, and rightly so. An "Iwuzgonna" is what an "I'magonna" changes into in the late fall. I wuzgonna fix that problem with the woodshed roof and Iwuzgonna get those willows out of the ditch...aaand about a year from now I suspect that changing the door on the shed will have become an Iwuzgonna. This winter is going to be the inception of a master plan...I'magonna make a list of all these minor chores and then just work off that list all summer, and I'magoona list them according to priority...the oldest Iwuzgonnas will be topmost Imagonnas and things should go smooth as cream, unlesssss...the winter I'magonna turns into a spring Iwuzgonna.

October 30, 1985

THINKING BIG
...but smaller is more restfull

Y'know, I think one of my big problems with going through this life is that I don't think big enough....I just plain have trouble thinking big. F'rinstance, the other day some of us were talking about this and that and nothing in particular when one of the guys asked me what I'd do with all the money if I won the Publisher's Clearing House Sweeps.

I told him I wasn't sure how much the 'sweeps' was going to pay, and he told me it was eleven million dollars. After I thought about it for a minute, I decided that I would take the money and have all the dents pounded out of my pickup and then get it painted....Yep, that's what I would like to do with all that money.

The guy said that wouldn't use up all the winnings orrr even come close to using it all. Well, I thought again and told him that I guessed I'd try to find some bucket seats for it...you know, scour the wrecking yards to find some real nifty bucket seats for my dear ol' pickup. Wow...! With all the dents gone and a new paint job and bucket seats, it would really be sumpthin'.

One of the other fells said that I must have the most expensive body and fender man in the business...either that or I just didn't relate to that much money. That was it alright, I just can't think that big.

Now, if the sweepstakes was eleven thousand dollars instead of eleven million, I could relate real good....Yeah, good relations there. That's within my scope of the financial world...I can understand that amount.

One of the other guys spoke up and said, "Lemmee tell ya a story about a boy in a small town in Alabama who they thought was pretty darn dumb. They would call him over and lay a dime and a nickel side by side and tell him he could have his choice. He would always take the nickel because it was the biggest coin. Time and time again he always took the nickel.

One day a stranger in town watched this lil' scenario taking place and when it was over and the boy had walked away, he stopped him and said, "Son, don't you know that dime is worth twice as much as a nickel?" The boy said, "Sure I do mister, a dime is ten cents and a nickel is five cents."

The man asked him, "Then why do you take the nickel?" The boy told him, "Mister, how many times would they play that game with me if I started takin' the dimes?" Now...there's a kid that could think big....He was lookin' way into the future for sure.

Anyhow, gettin' back to how I'd use up eleven million American bucks...I guess after I got my pickup all dolled up, I'd take the ELW (ever lovin' wife) on a trip from here to the East Coast drivin' the north route and then takin' the south route from the East Coast back home again, and I'd make sure that she didn't have to cook even one meal on the whole trip....We'd eat out all the time and stay at the best mediocre motels we could find on the route. That ought to just about use up the whole kit and kaboodle...by the time we had all the film processed.

Yep...I hafta start thinkin' a lot bigger.

Happy Leap Year to everyone, have a great one!

January 10, 1996

THE JOYS OF THE PHYSICAL CHECKUP

A sure-fire way to achieve real sickness.

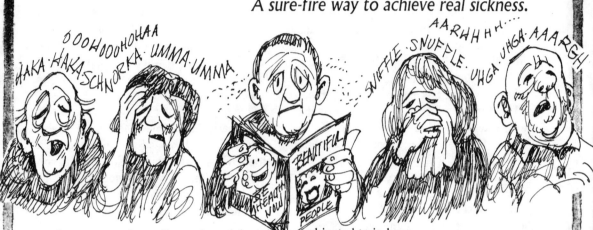

I guess we've all read articles in magazines at one time or another that say, "Eat right, get plenty of rest, and get regular physical checkups"...well, I figured that one out of three wasn't too bad so, let's get a checkup...make an appointment with a well-equipped clinic and get the ol' carcass looked at.

Well, after getting into the reception room a half hour early, the girl gives out this clipboard with a questionnaire that looks like a pre-med final exam. After filling in all the blanks and putting check marks in the little boxes and handing it to the desk, the girl says, "And just what is the nature of your illness...?" After explaining there is no illness and getting an odd look from everyone in the room, the girl says, "Take a seat, the doctor has a lot of sick people to see first."

After thumbing through some very ancient magazines, the eyes start roaming around the room...everyone in there is coughing or holding his head or somebody else's head and you begin to worry about what kind of horrible disease you might be subjected to in here.

About an hour past the time of the appointment another girl comes out with another list of questions and a little bottle with a napkin wrapped around it (poor disguise) and takes a double shot of blood out of the very best vein she can find...you get on the scales and she says, "Tch-tch-tch." shaking her head and then takes out the ol' blood pressure kit and pumps it up till your arm feels like it belongs on Popeye the Sailor, she then orders you back into the waiting room which has even sicker people in it now, some seem to be writhing with extreme fevers.

After about an hour of studying the intricate structure of the leaves on a too tall rubber tree in a redwood tub, the long awaited words, "Doctor will see you now" come ringing through the room and you're taken to a cubicle where the only thing to sit on is a hard cold table...another long wait until the doctor comes in and asks all the same questions over again and sends you down for a bunch of x-rays and more blood is donated to another collector, then you are ordered back to the waiting room again...it's not so full this time, a lot of them must have died.

Finally, back in the cubicle, the doctor says, "I can't seem to find any reason for your being here....You seem perfectly healthy." After explaining about how I thought a checkup was a good idea (another odd look) he asks again if I was sure I wasn't holding something back that he should know about.

He was right...I was holding back telling him about how I took a day off work (no pay), drove 85 miles, sat around in a room that reminded me of a leper colony, nothing to eat for hours, and weak from loss of blood. I was not ready to listen to how valuable his time was...while sitting in his shop where he would be anyhow, but I didn't say any of that stuff.

Instead, I told him thanks for his time, said I was glad I was healthy, and left the place feeling like the orphan kid in "Oliver Twist" when he asked for a second bowl of gruel.

Then the bill came...real sickness settled in, think I'll just eat right and get plenty of rest...those checkups will ruin your health.

December 2, 1981

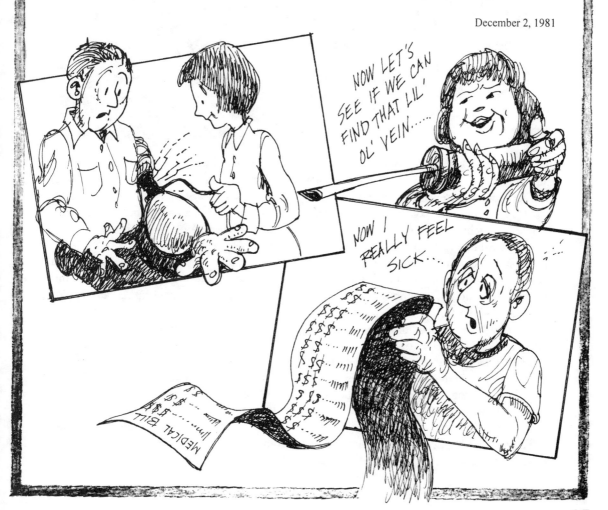

THE COOKWARE DEMONSTRATION (almost)

An unusual occupation, the home cookware salesman –
the trade had pretty much died out by the end of the 1950s

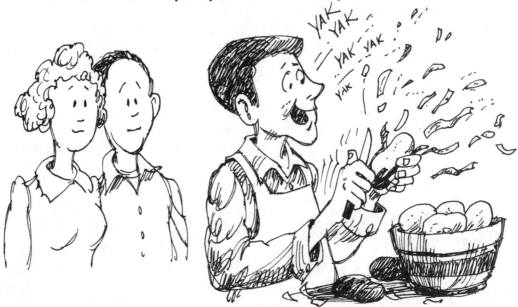

Wellll, the ELW (ever lovin' wife) went and did it....She bought a whole new set of kitchen cooking utensils, from the skillets right up through the pots and pans. The whole enchilada and everything matches...all one full blown set of cooking hardware. Now I'm afraid to even boil an egg for myself on those times when she isn't home...'fraid I'll scratch one of 'em or break a handle off.

It brought to mind the first set of cooking ware that we bought when we were just fresh married kids. The stuff was all aluminum wear and featured waterless cooking. I think it was called by the brand name of Wearever, and we used it for a long time.

The way we happened to buy that set in the first place was after a salesman called

us and talked us into letting him come and demonstrate the great Wearever cookware. This was in 1949 and we were living on the Forest Service compound in Callahan, where I was gainfully employed at the time.

The fella showed up agreeably to appointment and brought in a big box full of stuff...pots and pans, potatoes, apples and an apron for himself. He talked a steady stream about how he was gonna make us applesauce, boiled potatoes and do it all without adding one drop of water or anything except seasoning.

We couldn't get a word in edgewise he talked so darn fast. The apple peelings were flyin' and the potato skin was commin' off as fast as he was talking. When he got ready to start cookin' he asked where the range was, and I thought he meant the summer pasture so I just got started tellin' him, and he almost shouted at me, "No, no...the cooking range, the stove you cook on!"

The ELW pointed to our cook stove, which came with the house we were living in, and the poor guy went white and pale. I thought he was gonna faint, and he blurted out, "That's a wood cook stove! I've never cooked anything on a wood cook stove. Oh gosh! What am I gonna do?"

This was great, the ELW and I were in command now and we took over with style and grace...doing everything without water just the way he said.

By golly, you know what? That was great applesauce, and the spuds were really delicious. As we sat there eating this food with the now deflated salesman, we decided to buy his cookware. He wasn't a bad fella once he got off his super sales delivery, and we enjoyed his visit.

We still have some of the remains of that set....It was good stuff, but everything has a predetermined length of usefulness and then PHTTT!

November 9, 1994

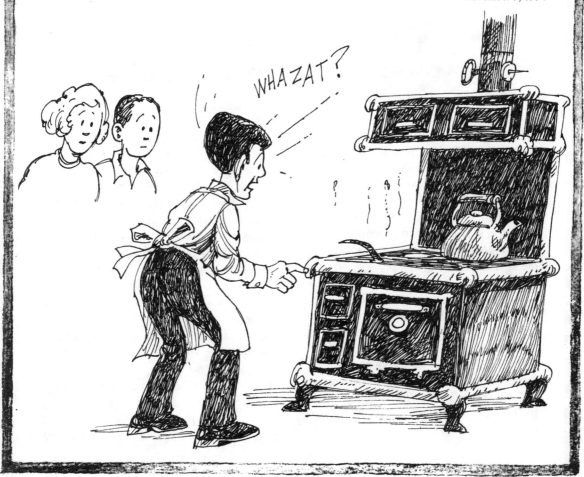

SAD STORIES OF THE "GOOD OL' DAYS"

...and other questionable memories

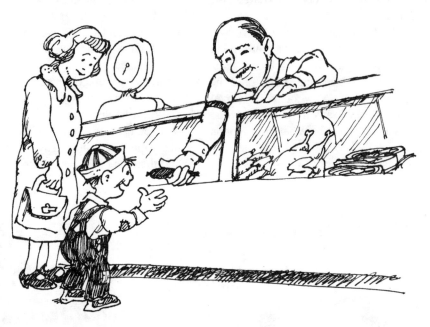

I'm not saying we should return to the "good ol' days" mind you, but it's kind of neat every once in awhile to remember some of the stuff that went on then.

F'rinstance, remember when you went shopping the butcher's shop, and he always gave the kids a slice of weenie? Just a small token, but it sure went over big with the kids...and the parents too.

The bakery shops had a unwritten rule of public relationship....When you bought a dozen cookies, he would toss in an extra one making it 13...a "baker's dozen" so the term said.

Remember when you bought a pair of shoes, the store gave you a shoehorn...a shiny metal one with the store's name or the brand of shoes stamped on it. (What's a shoehorn, daddy?)

Remember how guys would sit around and tell "poor stories?" you know...like, "When I was a kid we were so poor that..." One of my all time favorites was, "Our family was so poor that our clothes were real tattered rags....When my brother and I would run in the wind, they'd hum."

When we'd get new shoes for Christmas we saved the boxes they came in. The cardboard would be good for cutting out insoles to patch the holes that would happen. Shoebox cardboard was real tough material in those days...almost waterproof too.

Another one was, "Us kids were so skinny that we had to run around in the shower or we wouldn't get wet"...orrr, "We were so skinny that Mom had to put the stopper in the shower stall to keep us from going down the drain"...aaand, "We were so poor that we ate dried apples for breakfast, drank water for lunch and swelled up for dinner"....Pretty drab diet.

"Hand-me-down clothes" were a fact of growing up...the oldest kid in the family got clothes passed to him from a cousin or somebody, and when he outgrew 'em they went down to little brother and so on until they were beyond mending, but there were always fresh ones coming down the line.

I use to wonder who the lucky guy was way up the line that got the brand new clothes...the first timers.

During one of these sessions on braggin' about how poor they were as kids, a fella over in the shadows spoke for the first time and said, "You guys don't know how lucky you were....I was the only boy in our family." That kind of explained why he was a little bit different from the rest of the guys. I'll bet he had a tough time growing up and going to school an' everything in that situation.

One last one (finally) and then I'll quit (Oh boy!)...."When we were kids Dad couldn't afford the 15 cents for haircuts, so every spring he'd just set fire to it, and we'd start fresh." Come on you guys...enough already. (Hurray!)

October 18, 1995

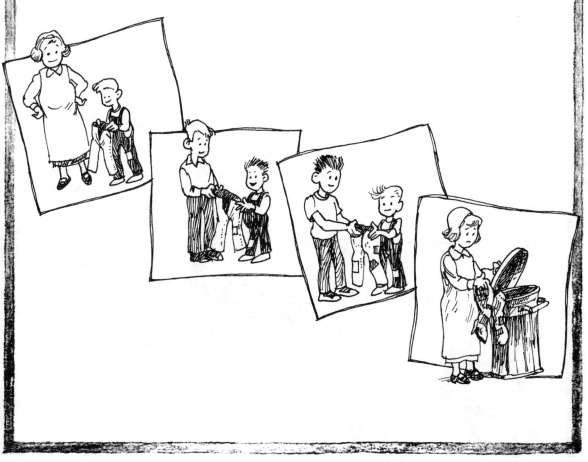

A FLYING FOREST SERVICE ADVENTURE
first class or coach - all the same

Y'know, with all these forest fires going on this season it causes me to recall a few of my experiences when I worked for the USFS out of the Callahan station...that was B.B.C. (before barber college) of course. I remember one fire experience, it may have been the one that caused me to consider going into another line of work. It was the summer of 1949 and we hadn't had one fire in this district all season.

The Callahan station was in the Scott District of the Shasta Forest in those days and we had acquired the nickname "Ironpants" because we had very few fires and no big ones at all. Because of this we were sent out of our district to other fires since there was no immediate need for all of us (four man team) to be on hand constantly.

In August of that year I was sent to a fire on the Stanislaus National Forest. One man from McCloud, one from Mt. Shasta and me from Callahan. We were to

catch a plane ride from Mott Field near Dunsmuir and fly to Columbia where there was supposed to be an airfield long enough to accommodate the old Ford Tri-Motor airplane in the hot weather and high altitude.

The old Tri-Motor was sitting there waiting for us and we got aboard the old corrugated aluminum air ship to find that it had just come from an assignment where they had been dropping supplies to a fire camp. The inside of the fuselage had no seats, hay was strewn all over from the bales that had been dropped to the pack stock and there was no door...only a wooden bar across the door opening. The co-pilot had to hand prop all three engines by standing on a rickety wooden step ladder...one at a time they all started okay.

The pilot flew the old concrete compass (highway 99) at the breakneck speed of 78 MPH indicated. Looking down at the traffic on the hiway we noticed that hay

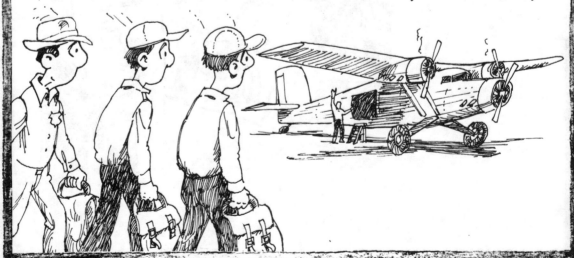

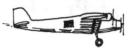

trucks were passing us up like we were parked. When the plane got over the town of Sacramento the pilot took a new heading to the south east and followed a barely paved road toward Sonora.

He circled around until he located an air strip where he figured the town of Columbia should be and he remarked, "Wow! that looks kinda short for this ol' bird." Just about then the co-pilot noticed an old C-47 (DC-3 Dakota?) just off the runway and he said, "If that guy got in there we sure can." So down we went. The guy did a nice job of it, we landed a little short and just as the manzanita brush and boulders were looming up in front he cranked in brakes and left rudder...ground bound safe and sound.

We got our gear and walked over to the hangar where there was a truck waiting to take us to the fire camp...one of the "hangar bums" said, as we walked by, "Y'know, that's the biggest plane we ever

seen land here." The fellow from Mt. Shasta, who was an ex paratrooper from WW-2, said, "Oh yeah? What about that C-47 sittin' there?...the guy said, "Oh that belongs to the F.B.O. here. He bought that at an auction down in Livermoore a few months ago. It doesn't fly so he hadda take the wings and engines off and truck it up here, then put it back together. He thinks he's gonna get 'er flyin' someday."

We found out later that the Tri-Motor waited until the next morning and was able to take off by not refueling and used up every last foot of runway. After the fire duty they flew us back to Mott in a Stinson Voyager...much better trip...the engine even had a starter on it and there were doors on an' everything. In June of the following year (1950) I enrolled in Barber College...the same year I was offered year round employment with the Forest Service. A tough decision. I'll never know if I chose the best route or not.

August 3, 1994

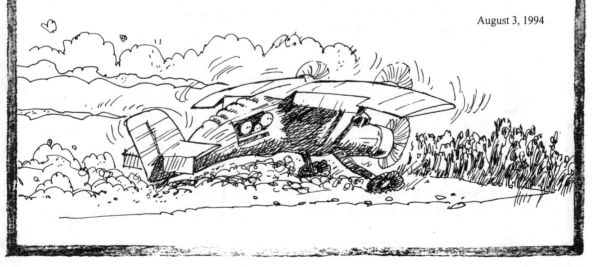

HOT PEPPERS.....EEEYOWWWW!

a sure cure for plugged sinuses

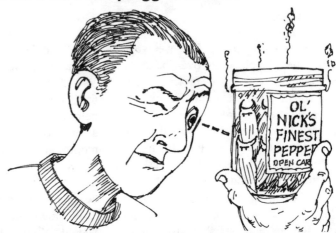

Sometimes I wonder if the whole country west of the Rockies hasn't gone berserk on the "Hot Pepper Mania," or whatever you wish to call it. What I mean is, it seems like almost all fast food joints and eatery type cafes these days offer an "ortega this" or a "jallapeno that," or a "chili whatchacallit" on the menu.

Cheese companies offer a jallapeno type cheese...little green specks in these with a lot of authority...whew! There's "ortega burgers" and chili pepper omelets" and so on. Personally, I can't figure out what it is that makes us want to torture our innards with all this heat...but I like it, I just can't help it, I like it and as long as they keep on making Rolaids and stuff like that, I will probably keep on eating that kind of junk.

Maybe, in my case anyway, it stems from the days when my dad and I used to try to out heat each other with hot peppers and all sorts of chili peppers. About every time we would get together for a meal at either his home or mine, we would each trot out a jar of hot peppers or some sort of

hot pickled vegetables to try on each other.

We'd no sooner get the roast carved or the steaks served when it became time for the old ritualistic game of "I can stand 'em hotter than you can," and my memory of those occasions are very dear to me...sort of an off road game of chicken.

The first one that allowed tears to stream from the eyes or ran for a drink of water was considered the loser and the other fella would have the pleasure of saying, in a cool type of delivery, "Whazz-amatter, too warm for ya?"

Now, those jars of hot pickled wax peppers, cauliflower, carrots etc., that you see in the stores were one thing...they were tolerable, plenty hot alright but not destructive to living tissue. We were always on the lookout for a new brand of pickled hot peppers...red peppers, green peppers, short peppers or long peppers, as long as they were hot peppers.

On one of my dad's winter trips down to the state of Arizona or New Mexico, or some place like that, he brought back a jar of real mean looking peppers and the game began...dad said, "I want you to try these peppers, they are about the finest I ever came across."

I looked at that jar and I could almost see those lil' short fat peppers in there leering at me and I could almost hear them saying, "Come on sucker, try one!"

Well sir, this time the dinner was at my house and the ELW (ever lovin' wife) had a top notch pot roast for dinner and dad set those peppers right on the table in front of me. I think he had been conditioning himself with the darn things 'cause he took a pretty healthy chunk and looked me right in the eye so I could see he wasn't tearing up.

My turn....I took a little larger piece than he did...COWABUNGA!! Instant pain along with some other interesting side effects. The eyes watered up, the ears began to get this humming noise in 'em and sweat was forming on the eyelids and in back of the neck...then the vision went, everything got blurry.

I had been soundly defeated. I lost all my cool, couldn't help gasping for breath and I had to turn down his offer of seconds.

I truly believe my teeth were soft for two weeks and I couldn't make a fist or whistle...but, y'know, I cherish the memory of that evening and how proud my dad was that I had waved the white flag...finally.

November 8, 1989

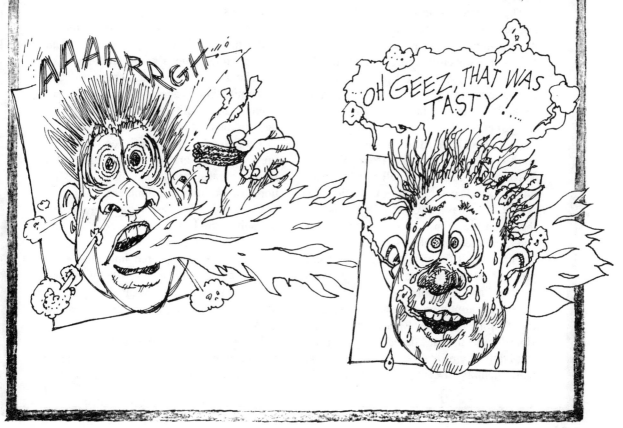

HOT PEPPERS AGAIN
...and another "eating on the road" adventure

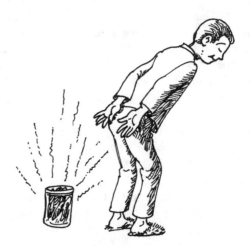

The response to last week's effort about hot pepper experiences has been overwhelming...puhleez, no more hot peppers, although I sincerely appreciate all the lil' incendiary critters that I've received. I have to award the "Most Attention Getting Award" to Jack and Jane Berggreen....Whew!!

Talk about heat! They made them from fresh jalalpeno peppers from Yakima, Washington, and I can tell you they are gonna save me a lot of wood this winter...all I have to do is take the lid off the jar and set it in the middle of the room and keep a respectable distance.

Through all the heat though, there is a mighty fine taste that comes through...very delicious and well done.

I have had numerous requests to extend the "Eating on the Road Away From Home" column that I dared to try...and the Boss dutifully printed, soooo, I'll offer one more memory of eating at cafes along the highways.

The truckers have very colorful nicknames for these lil' food ruiners along the concrete ribbons of our country...like, "Choke 'n Puke" and another one is "Gag 'n Vomit," but I have never found any that even came close to matching the descriptions...at least not that graphic.

There is one cafe experience that stands out in my memory that I will relate. We were on vacation and heading home just north of Calimesa in Southern California, the kids were with us, and we saw a cafe on a little knoll and decided to stop for a sandwich or something.

As soon as we entered into that damp, swamp cooler atmosphere, I knew we had made a mistake and I wanted to run, but the kids wanted a snack, soooo, what the heck.

You could tell the cook and the waitress had been having a fight, he was glaring over the steamy grill at her and she was sticking her tongue out at him. Our food (??) was slammed down in front of us, sodas sloshed over etc.

We finished whatever it was and I asked the waitress (Cinderella's stepmother) if I could have a dish of vanilla ice cream...she disappeared behind the counter and bent over the freezer, scooped up two helpings of vanilla and tossed it at me as she pranced by the table.

I thought it was the richest vanilla ice cream I had ever seen...real deep bright yellow, and after I got the first spoonful in my mouth my taste buds went berserk.

It was margarine! Two big dippers of margarine! I called "Miss Warmth" over and told her what the stuff was and she replied it couldn't be margarine because they didn't keep margarine in the freezer.

About that time the cook and the dishwasher broke out in loud laughter...uncontrollable eye watering laughter. They had pulled a joke on the gal...set the margarine container in with the ice cream and removed the tub of vanilla.

She tore off her apron and ran out screaming profanities, the cook is in uncontrollable laughing convulsions and the dishwasher is hee-hawing his little pointed head off and I've got this coating of grease in my mouth.

By this time both kids and the ELW (ever lovin' wife) are tee-heeing and guffawing all over the place; I'm the only one not having a real good time.

The cook came out and took the check and the money and says, "Just leave the tip on the table, I'll see that she gets it, an y'all have a good trip now, y'heah."....another pleasant "dining out" experience.

November 15, 1989

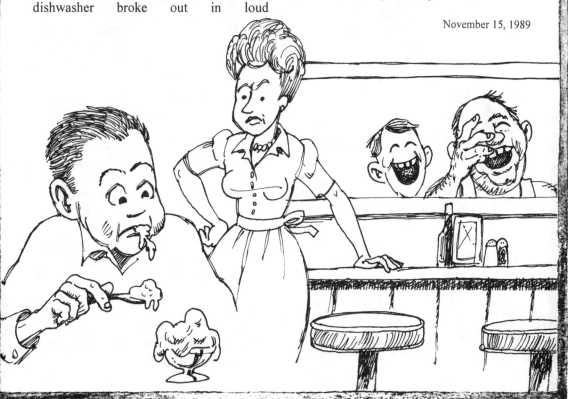

103

INFLATION

depressing thoughts for depression years kids

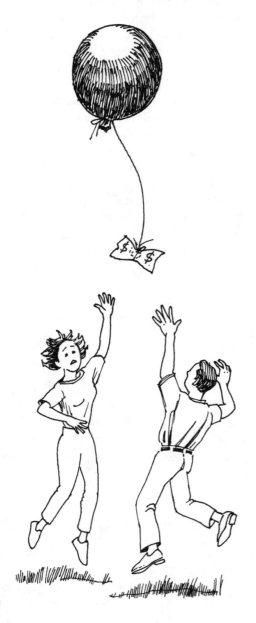

I am not the person in our house who does the shopping and buying very often. The ELW (ever lovin' wife) does the most of that sort of thing. I will pick up a few items at the store if I can work from a list, nothing heavy, just a few everyday type things that the home runs short of.

This is why I am not up on the way stuff has increased in price over the years....I have trouble with adapting to the rise. I keep thinking I'm back in the olde tymes with those prices that I first became acquainted with as a mere child.

F'rinstance, when I finally made it to the seventh grade in school (a lot of my relatives lost money on bets when I did) the gym coach asked me if I wanted to try out for some of the sports activities...he thought I had potential. I kind of liked the idea and I told him I would sure like to try.

He told me I would have to get a pair of tennis shoes and an athletic supporter. I told him I wouldn't have any trouble gettin' supporters...my dad and all my uncles really liked sports, but the tennis shoes might be a problem if they cost very much.

I had some money that I had earned from working in the hay that summer so I went to the store that sold these items. The tennis shoes were black and white high tops and cost $2.75 and that other thing cost 89 cents (yeah, I found out what it was) for a total of $3.64...almost a week's wages at 75 cents a day.

Now, ordinarily when the ELW and I are shopping and it's time to check out at the register, she will find something for me to do away from the area so I can't see the numbers of the total sale when they come up...she's afraid I'll get hit with the "big one" and fall over in a lifeless state...a bit over protective.

Anyhow, I have seen a lot of guys around lately who are at least as old as I am, wearing these new fangled tennis shoes that look like they would be real comfortable. You know, something to knock around in when we go over to the coast or to the great "Sin City" of Reno.

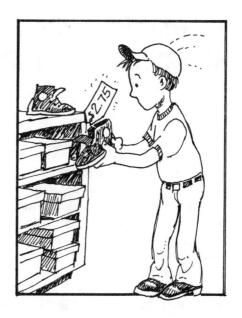

The next time we went to town the ELW shoved me into a shoe store for some these "squeak stop" tennys. I tried some on and by golly, they were light and soft...seemed to fit good and felt like they gave good support, so I told the guy I would take 'em.

When we got up the check out register he started to work me into the idea of buying some socks and other things, but I was too clever for him...I told him I had other socks at home besides the ones I was wearing. As he rang up the sale he said that I was real lucky because these shoes were ordinarily $39.99 but were on sale for $36.99.

The last words echoed through my ears like they were coming from far far away, "thirty nyun - nyun - nyun nyunnnn,"...my chest hurt, my eyes got hot, I felt cold and sweaty...this was surely the "big one."

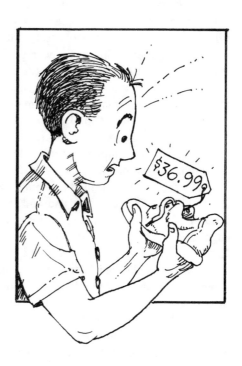

Tennis shoes? $36.99? You gotta be kidding! I can understand $189.99 for cowboy boots, but tennys for almost $37?

I think the ELW is gonna get me a set of total black-out blinders and earplugs to be installed when at, or near, the check out stands...a Father's Day gift that will keep on giving.

June 21, 1989

A CALL TO BRING BACK
HENRY FORD'S MODEL A

The other day while I had the hood of the car up...I was filling the little container that holds the windshield wiper cleanser, which is about the only thing I know how to do under the hood anymore...I was just casting an eye over the maze of wires and contraptions in there, wondering where the spark plugs were, if indeed there were spark plugs, and I thought it might be a good idea to check the water in the battery and check the oil.

The battery doesn't have caps on it and you don't add water to the battery...it was filled at the factory I was told. Ooooohkay, when I finally found the dip stick to check the engine oil level it turned out to be the stick for the transmission, there's a whole essay of information engraved on that little strip of metal.

The dip to check the oil in the crankcase turned up on the complete wrong side of the engine...clear on the other side from the filler cap. When I pulled the thing out it was about three feet long and had two bends in it with a lot of words along the edge...some of them said, "Full Level Hot," and some said, "Full Level Cold."

Since the engine had been shut off for about 20 minutes I figured it was about luke warm and there was no mark that said, "Luke Warm," so I gave up on checking the oil. I'm not even sure just exactly how much of that junk in there is engine and how much is accessory stuff.

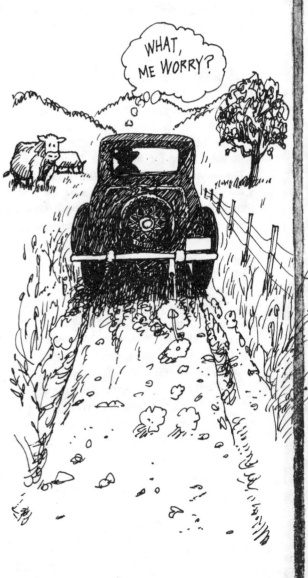

WHAT, ME WORRY?

I finally admitted to myself that the car is a complete mystery and should be left alone by a novice...my good ol' pickup and I still have a going relationship though, so I went over and lifted up the hood on it and gave myself an oral quiz on what and where everything was. I think I passed with about a 72 percent grade.

When we were kids we used to give old cars that we owned, a thing we called an "Okie Overhaul." We'd drain the gas, oil and water out of it, lay down about four old used tires on one side and push the car over on it's side so it would come to rest on the old tires.

With the car laying on it's side it was all stand up work...pull the pan off on one side, and if you had to, pull the head off from the other side, aaaand two guys could pass the tools back and forth without bending over.

By cutting out strips of bacon rind and laying them in the rod and main bearing caps and then with "armstrong torque"

we'd cinch those caps back on. This would give another five to six hundred miles before the engine would start knocking and rapping again...that is, if you kept plenty of second hand fifty weight motor oil in the crankcase and didn't push it too hard in the speed envelope.

Gas was expensive, about 12 cents a gallon, but we could stretch that by adding kerosene and a little ether with the gas...amazing performance.

Well, thank heaven for progress. These days in our present lil' Detroit miracles, if we break down we have to wait for somebody to come along who has a computer type diagnostic machine along with a ton of parts...aaannd who can say how many of those guys come along, say frinstance, in the Joshua Tree National Monument or in the Mojave Desert...today's motorists definitely have cleaner fingernails...as well as today's mechanics.

April 12, 1989

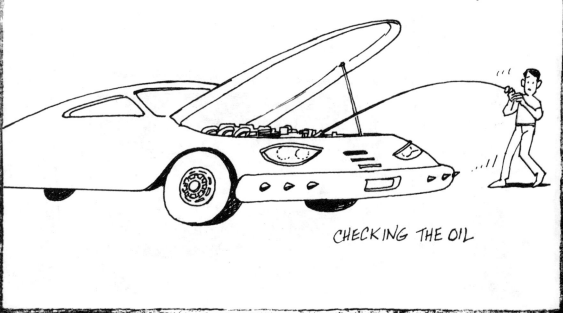

CHECKING THE OIL

IS THIS A GARAGE ...or a warehouse?

Mr. Webster, in his big book of words, says that the word "garage" means a shelter for automobiles, a business establishment where automobiles are stored or repaired, etc. Now, that sounds concise, simple and to the point doesn't it?

Well, then how come so many garages are chock full of stuff and the automobiles sit outside in the elements...sun, snow, rain, sleet and birds all taking a whack at the family carriage.

Most of our married life we have had a single car garage that became, in no time at all, a no car garage. That space that was built and designed for the family flivver became filled up with stuff like lawn mowers, table saws, boxes full of stored "valuables" etc. Later on we had what was called a car and a half garage...in no time at all it was transformed into a half a car garage and ultimately, a no car garage.

Stuff just takes over, it's spooky! The idea of parking the car in the barn after we have lost control of the garage just does not work too well. The barn is filled with all kinds of birds, owls, chickens and even a horse once in awhile...instant dirt and spot treatments.

The garage I have now was built the way I wanted it, at least as close to what I wanted that the ol' wallet would allow. It's a two car garage with a nice big work bench and storage at one end. Right after it was finished it looked big enough to house the Queen Mary with room left over for a PT boat or two.

Pretty quick a lot of space was lost to tools, cans full of various nuts, bolts, springs etc. Lawn mowers, cement mixers, spare lumber and old discarded electric motors and other "save-um" stuff. The walls began closing in from hanging stuff on nails along the sides.

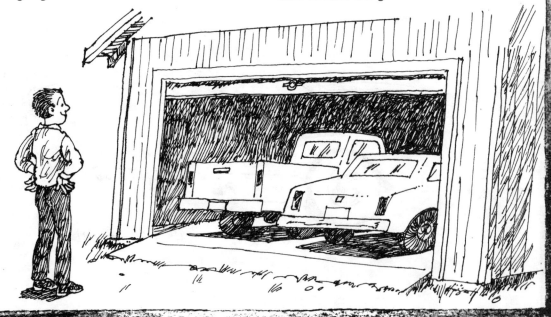

108

The ceiling became a planked deck with all sorts of goodies piled up there...stuff like old hand crank ice cream makers, old bamboo fly rods and fishing baskets, stuff that they don't even make anymore. Cartons of left over floor tile from various room remodelings.

I can still get the family sedan in there and also my very faithful pickup but somehow it seems like I have to squeeze along the sides after I get out of the car and shut the door...the garage is shrinking! Oh No!

I'm very careful to not leave the car or the pickup out of the garage for more than a week at a time, actually I put the vehicles inside each and every night, but sometimes we are away on a trip for almost a week.

While we are gone I sometimes get this sudden nervous attack..."Geez, what if we get home and there's no room in the garage for the car anymore?"

I'm convinced that our "stuff" is capable of taking over all available space in the garage thereby squeezing out the cars and pickups for which it was originally intended. The extra space in there seems to be shrinking much faster since the Greenview dump is closed.

Ya gotta haul all this metal stuff clear to Yreka now and that is the very category of stuff that wants my spare space....I have to watch it every minute and keep putting the vehicles away as often as possible to keep dibs on the space in there.

April 17, 1989

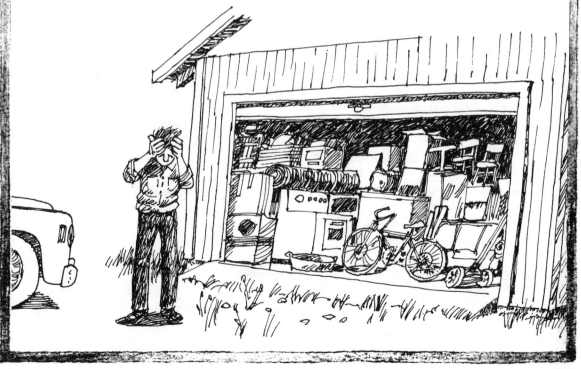

MEMORIES
no money - but good times

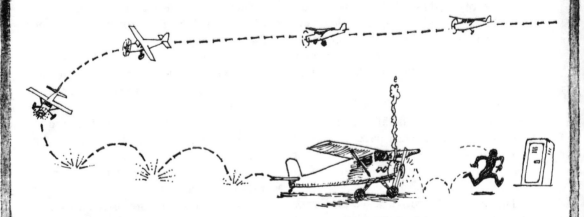

I read that some of the sure signs of aging are; you install a compass in your car, your fondest dreams are about prunes and you constantly think and talk about, "the old days." They left out one sign and that would be that you become a victim of a "short bladder range."

I just recently installed a compass in my car so I'm guilty of the first symptom. I didn't have it long though. It sprang a leak and all the fluid dripped out onto the dashboard and the little ball with degrees painted on it just fell to the dry bottom of the dry enclosure, never to rotate again. I have since replaced it with a new one. Gotta have a compass. Why? You ask? I don't know.

So far I've not had any dreams about prunes and I'm gonna knock on wood with that one. I know one fella who says he has dreams about Metamucil, but he's a little more sophisticated than most senior citizens and he has more money too.

Talking about the old days is one I'll confess to. I enjoy some of the experiences that I had in the old days. F'rinstance, the thing that comes to mind is the holiday that we just had. The Fourth of July. I can remember some awesome Fourth of July picnics that were held at the Scott Mountain Campground. Space up there was staked out and claimed by some member of the group a day or two ahead of time so there would be the choicest part of the area reserved. Room in the meadow for a baseball game and a shady place for the food...and there was a huge bunch of food. Even during the lean years of the late 1930s there was always plenty of food. Chicken, salads, homemade rolls and melon. Somehow there was always ice cream for the kids. Money was pooled and the grown-ups said, "We gotta get those kids some ice cream." It was shipped to Cap Farrington's store in gallon containers and packed in big insulated bags. Three gallons to a bag.

Now those are what I call fond

memories, those days before World War Two. Nobody had much money (especially around these parts) but we sure enjoyed living.

As for that "short bladder range" affliction. I used to hear a lot of fascinating stories about that problem when I was flying a lot. Three pound Hills Brothers coffee cans were very much in demand but not practical when mixed company was aboard. Just think what a difficult chore it is to land an airplane with your legs crossed. I heard of one guy who actually declared an emergency in order to get landing preference ahead of the other traffic.

Military airplanes during WW-2 had "relief tubes" installed in the cockpit. Once in awhile when the ground crew would have a spat with the pilot they would plug the relief tube. A very mean thing to do to a pilot, especially if the airplane was inverted during a dogfight in combat.

Oh well, I guess when you consider the alternative to growing old it's not so bad to have a couple of those symptoms show up.

July 7, 1999

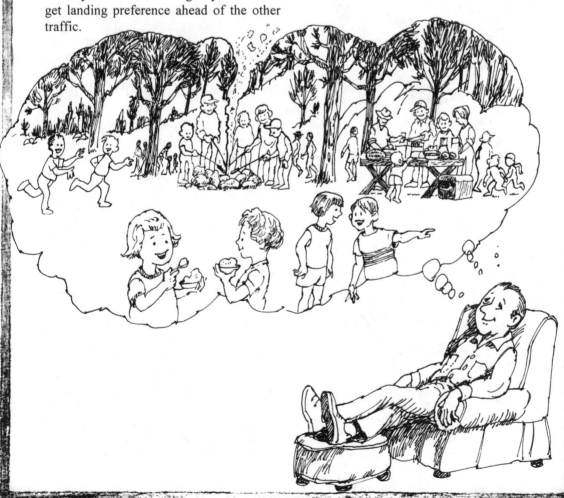

VALENTINES DAY AT SCHOOL
...and the horrors thereof

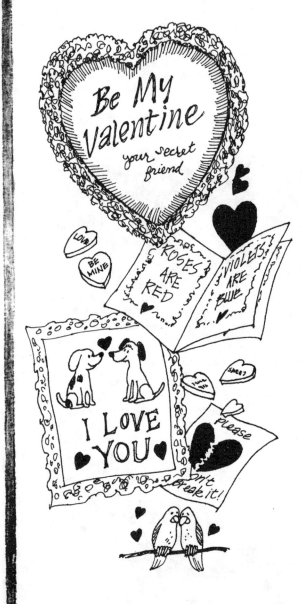

With St. Valentine's Day coming upon us, as it does each and every year, I'm reminded of this event and how it was conducted in the grammar school that I attended...and attended, and attended, and attended. It always seemed to turn out to be some sort of an underhanded popularity contest. I didn't realize it at the time, but looking back on it that's what it was alright. It's only taken me some 50 plus years to have this dawn upon me....I learn slow but once I get it, I forget it right away.

For about a week before Valentine's Day the teacher would rig up this barrel in the classroom, get it all decorated up with red and white tissue paper and little red hearts pasted all over it. On top there was a lid with only a slit in it large enough to drop a small card or envelope through. The idea was to drop a Valentine in there to one of the class cuties. I think you could buy those small Valentine cards for about 10 cents a dozen back there in the dark ages, so it wasn't a heavy financial caper. The lil' girls would drop in cards for certain little boys and lil' boys would drop in cards to the girl of his choice. You could look around the room and see guys leaning over their desk covering up the card with one hand and writing with the other one so no one else could see who's name he was writing on the card - then slip over to the barrel and drop it in.

The girls were different about it. I think they must have put the name on and signed the cards at home and then slipped 'em in the barrel when there was nobody in the classroom, orrr sumpthin' like that cause you could never catch 'em in the act of droppin' the card in there.

The teacher must have had a heart in her someplace because she would buy a few cards and have them laid back for some of the poor lil' boys and girls who wouldn't get cards from anybody in the class.

Well, finally the big day would arrive...the day to crack open that barrel and hand out all the cards to the kids. The teacher would call the name of the recipient and the kid would go up in the front of the room and get each card as she called it. Two or three of the cuter and more popular girls would be gathering up quite a stack of cards and about the same number of boys who were very popular would begin piling them up on their desk. Geez! Here we were, just lil' ol' kids in the third or fourth grade getting our first lumps in the cruel, cold world of a sort of popularity contest.

Well, finally it was over and all the kids were arranging their cards on their desk and enjoying looking at them...it amounted to quite a stack of Valentines cause there was about 30 kids in the class. Somehow or other I came up with two Valentines...one of them was signed, "from your friend," in a handwriting that was very adult looking...just like the teacher's writing - what a coincidence - some lil' girl with handwriting just like the teachers. The other one was from a kid named James....I looked across the room and there was James smiling at me. We always used to sort of wonder about James, but what the heck...a card is a card. Happy Valentine's Day to all.

February 8, 1989

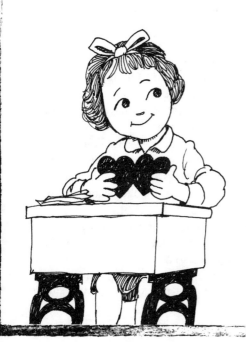
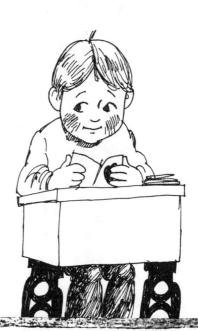

AFTER ELW *(ever lovin' wife)*

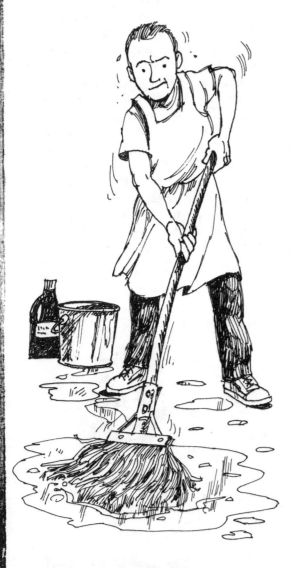

You know, this bachelor life is something I've never experienced before, oddly enough.

I was a student in my second year of high school living at home, of course, with my mom taking care of me, when I quit school to join the Army (ours) because I was afraid the "fun" would be over if I waited until I finished school. It could well have taken 15 years for me to graduate at the rate I was going. Anyhow, being in the Army was sure not a bachelor's life. Your platoon became your family.

After the war I enrolled in junior college and shared a room in the "GI Bill Arms" just off campus with another ex-GI Still not alone. From there I was married and for 49 ½ years. I had everything done for me and was spoiled rotten by a wonderful lady who was my wife, lover, companion, and mother of my children.

Now, all of a sudden I am a bachelor, and it's on-the-job training.

I ran into a friend of mine the other day, and he, after a few minutes said, "Wow! Buzz, that's great after shave lotion you're wearing. What is it?" I told him it wasn't after shave lotion. It was Lemon Pledge.

I had been catching up on learning the woes of dusting and cleaning furniture, and I used Lemon Pledge because it made stuff shine as well as clean.

He mentioned he might get some and try it for under arm deodorant 'cause he liked the fragrance so much.

Last week I had an appointment with my dermatologist in Medford. We always visit a little while before he gets to his duties. During our little chat he happened to glance at my boots and said, "That's a real nice shine on those boots, Buzz. What do you use?"

I told him that I didn't use shoe polish and explained that I must have splashed some Mop and Glo on 'em when I was doing the kitchen floor. It's a kind of linoleum cleaner that leaves a shine after it cleans and dries.

A pal of mine dropped over one evening and we sat in the kitchen to chat. He said to me, "Well Buzz, it looks like you're a pretty good housekeeper. At least the sink isn't full of dirty dishes, and there aren't a bunch of dirty pots and pans on the stove." I told him that I don't use dishes or pots and pans, just silverware and Styrofoam cups.

I just make a sandwich out of everything and lean over the sink to eat it. Then all you have to do is rinse the crumbs down the drain. Of course, Jello is kind of tough to keep between the bread slices. It keeps wiggling out.

Running the washing machine is one thing I've got a handle on from all those years of towels from the shop.

Now, ironing is another story. A lady asked me how I got that big damaged spot on my index finger. I told here it was from testing the iron to see if it was hot. It was! Thanks for the wash-and-wear stuff.

Mending and sewing, you ask? Noooo prob. They make duct tape in colors now.

June 10, 1998

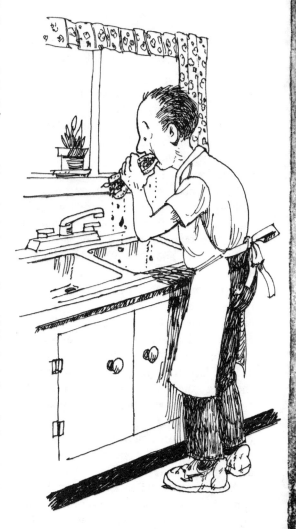

115

THE FEMININE TOUCH

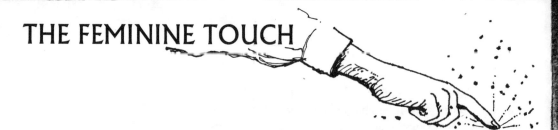

Y'know, studying the grocery shelves these days makes me think the food companies are designing their efforts to accommodate the bachelor population. There are so many foods on the shelves that require only the minimum of know-how to get ready for the table. I have to say though, these one and two step preparations lose something in the flavor and excitement of foods that are prepared with loving hands and a know-how cook. They will get a fella over the boredom of fixing the same ol' corned beef hash five nights a week and a couple of Ho-Hos for dessert.

If it weren't for the microwave and frozen foods it would not be so easy though. Those TV dinners are really not all that bad anymore. There have been some definite improvements in those items in the last few years. I find myself checking the instructions on the TV dinners to make sure they can be nuked. I just hate heating up the oven anymore when the stuff can be put in the microwave and be done faster and less mess than with the oven.

Case in point. For as long as I can remember angel food cake has been one of my most favorite desserts and I prefer them unfrosted. My mom used to make angel food cakes and it was quite a process. First she would gather up enough eggs and then separate the whites from the yolks very carefully and then proceed with the rest of the stuff that went with the egg whites and finally get it in the oven and wait for the thing to bake. I saw an angel food cake mix on the shelf in the store and the words that caught my attention said, "One Step Angel Food Cake Mix." I checked out the directions on the back of the box and it said just add one and a quarter cups of water to the mix, beat for two minutes, pour into pan and bake. I had no hope at all for this thing turning out to resemble a cake but I had to try because I had this terrible hunger for an angel food cake. By golly, I have to tell you that darn thing turned out pretty darn good and I have done several more since then. There is one thing that is better about this one step cake mix than making one from scratch, and that is you don't have to bake a yellow cake later on to get rid of the egg yolks that are left over from making the angel food. I was never a yellow cake fan. To me they always tasted like a rubber sponge with frosting on it. You could wash the car with a left over yellow cake so it wouldn't be a complete loss and waste of egg yolks.

Sadly though, there is no substitute for a feminine touch with the food in the kitchen. There has to be that good ol' know-how that makes home meals what they are when they are prepared right.

December 3, 1998

IN CLOSING...

I would like to leave you with this old blessing; it is still as meaningful in this new millennium as it was in the last...maybe more so.

May the Good Lord take a liking to you, may the wind be always to your back, and may you be in heaven a week before the devil finds out you have died.

Buzz

There you have it: 60 of Buzz's essays. They were fun to illustrate — as you can probably tell.

Buzz has written over 900 of these essays; so there must be 850 plus that could be illustrated and published yet. Since we have a whole new century to kick around in, perhaps we'll do a sequel......
......well, we'll see.

John

117

FOR ADDITIONAL COPIES

SEND ORDER TO:

SKETCHBOOK PRESS
P.O. BOX 220
FORT JONES, CA 96032-0220

"Once Over Lightly," ISBN 0-9700301-0-X, $15.95
California addresses add $1.16 sales tax (7.25%)
Shipping: $2.50 1st book, $1.25 each additional book

Also still available:
"Scott Valley Sketchbook," ISBN 0-9700301-1-8, $15.85
California addresses add $1.15 sales tax (7.25%)
Shipping: $2.50 1st book, $1.25 each additional book

ORDER FORM

Enclosed is $_____ for _____copies of Once Over Lightly

Enclosed is $_____ for _____copies of Scott Valley Sketchbook

Name_____

Address_____

City_____State_____ZIP_____

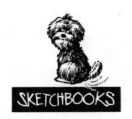